CW00958682

Continuity of Care in Breastfeeding: Best Practices in the Maternity Setting

Karin Cadwell, PhD, RN, FAAN, IBCLC
The Healthy Children Project
The Center for Breastfeeding
East Sandwich, Massachusetts

Cindy Turner-Maffei, MA, IBCLC
The Healthy Children Project
The Center for Breastfeeding
East Sandwich, Massachusetts

JONES AND BARTLETT PUBLISHERS
Sudbury, Massachusetts
BOSTON   TORONTO   LONDON   SINGAPORE

World Headquarters
Jones and Bartlett Publishers
40 Tall Pine Drive
Sudbury, MA 01776
978-443-5000
info@jbpub.com
www.jbpub.com

Jones and Bartlett Publishers
Canada
6339 Ormindale Way
Mississauga, Ontario L5V 1J2
CANADA

Jones and Bartlett Publishers
International
Barb House, Barb Mews
London W6 7PA
UK

Jones and Bartlett's books and products are available through most bookstores and online booksellers. To contact Jones and Bartlett Publishers directly, call 800-832-0034, fax 978-443-8000, or visit our website, www.jbpub.com.

The authors, editor, and publisher have made every effort to provide accurate information. However, they are not responsible for errors, omissions, or for any outcomes related to the use of the contents of this book and take no responsibility for the use of the products and procedures described. Treatments and side effects described in this book may not be applicable to all people; likewise, some people may require a dose or experience a side effect that is not described herein. Drugs and medical devices are discussed that may have limited availability controlled by the Food and Drug Administration (FDA) for use only in a research study or clinical trial. Research, clinical practice, and government regulations often change the accepted standard in this field. When consideration is being given to use of any drug in the clinical setting, the health care provider or reader is responsible for determining FDA status of the drug, reading the package insert, and reviewing prescribing information for the most up-to-date recommendations on dose, precautions, and contraindications, and determining the appropriate usage for the product. This is especially important in the case of drugs that are new or seldom used.

Library of Congress Cataloging-in-Publication Data
Cadwell, Karin.
  Continuity of care in breastfeeding : best practices in the maternity setting / Karin Cadwell and Cindy Turner-Maffei.
    p. ; cm.
  Includes bibliographical references and index.
  ISBN-13: 978-0-7637-5184-5 (alk. paper)
  ISBN-10: 0-7637-5184-7 (alk. paper)
  1. Breastfeeding. 2. Continuum of care. I. Turner-Maffei, Cindy. II. Title.
  [DNLM: 1. Breast Feeding. 2. Continuity of Patient Care--organization & administration. 3. Evidence-Based Medicine. 4. Maternal-Child Nursing. WS 125 C126c 2009]
  RJ216.C2283 2009
  649'.33--dc22

                    2008003506

6048

Production Credits
Publisher: Kevin Sullivan
Aquisitions Editor: Emily Ekle
Aquisitions Editor: Amy Sibley
Editorial Assistant: Patricia Donnelly
Editorial Assistant: Rachel Shuster
Associate Production Editor: Amanda Clerkin
Associate Marketing Manager: Rebecca Wasley

Manufacturing and Inventory Control
  Supervisor: Amy Bacus
Composition: Shawn Girsberger
Cover Design: Kate Ternullo
Cover Image Credit: © David Kelly/Shutterstock, Inc.
Printing and Binding: Malloy, Inc.
Cover Printing: Malloy, Inc.

Printed in the United States of America
12 11 10 09 08   10 9 8 7 6 5 4 3 2 1

Contents

Acknowledgments

Between the two of us, we have more than 60 years experience working in the field of breastfeeding support. We are grateful for the many conversations, questions, debates, and discussions (some pretty heated!) we have had with healthcare workers, breastfeeding advocates, and supporters who candidly described to us their challenges and successes as they worked to achieve continuity of care in maternity care, medical practice, and community breastfeeding support settings. These conversations have inspired this book. Perhaps you don't remember your comment to one of us during the coffee break or over lunch at a conference, an elevator conversation, a discussion at a meeting, or during a consultation in person or by phone at your place of work, but you sparked the development of these ideas and our quest to seek doable solutions—our need to integrate and clarify our experiences and yours. Please know that you have our enduring thanks.

Thank you for challenging our assumptions. By getting to know you and your issues in many countries around the world, in practice settings and communities with different challenges and opportunities, we learned that there is no single solution, no easy fix in the implementation of optimal care for breastfeeding.

You have not only been willing to engage in the dialogue that allowed us to develop the ideas in this book; you have, by your example, allowed us to keep believing that it is possible to provide all mothers and babies with optimal breastfeeding care and support. Whenever discouragement and frustration loomed large, an unexpected updraft would come our way: "I tried your suggestion and it worked." "The quality team found the issue and we have succeeded in implementing skin-to-skin within a half-hour after birth." "This week we removed the pacifiers from all the carts. They are only available when indicated." "We finished training all the staff and our unnecessary supplementation rate is way down. Thank you for the help."

We also thank and remember the late James P. Grant, director of UNICEF from 1980 to 1995 and tireless advocate for children's health, who, together with his colleagues at UNICEF and the World Health Organization, inspired the international implementation of the Ten Steps to Successful Breastfeeding which now form the basis to the Baby-Friendly Hospital Initiative. The Ten Steps have provided us, and now more than 20,000 hospitals the world over, with an organizing framework for breastfeeding continuity of care.

Introduction

This book is an exploration of the impact of achieving continuity of care and optimal maternity care practices on breastfeeding outcomes. The material comes from our review of the literature and our experience in working with individual health workers, as well as hospitals and birth centers to improve breastfeeding outcomes. Much of this work has centered on helping maternity facilities to implement the WHO/UNICEF Ten Steps to Successful Breastfeeding, which form the basis of the Baby-Friendly Hospital Initiative.

In this book, we describe methods to achieve optimal breastfeeding initiation, duration, and exclusivity. The goals for the year 2010 in the U.S. are that breastfeeding rates will rise to (or above) 75% initiation, 50% duration at 6 months and 25% at 12 months. The goals for exclusive breastfeeding are 40% at 3 months and 17% at 6 months. While we are close to achieving our initiation goal, we are far from meeting the duration and exclusivity goals. Indeed, in the U.S. and many other countries a high percentage of breastfed babies leave the maternity setting having already consumed infant formula, typically not because of medical indications, but due to the impact of poor breastfeeding practices, lack of continuity of care or inadequate staff education. Every country and every hospital has unique barriers to achieving optimal care of the breastfeeding mother and her baby.

Exclusive breastfeeding, meaning giving no food or drink other than mother's milk to babies, is the style of infant feeding most highly associated with optimal infant and maternal health. If we are to achieve our goals for exclusive breastfeeding, maternity care practices must be a major focus.

Continuity of obstetric, maternity, and pediatric care is an essential component of maternal child health. This book focuses only on the maternity care practice setting. While maternity care practices occur during a short time period, recent research indicates that the experiences the mother and baby encounter around the time of birth have critical effect on the development of the mother/baby relationship, including the success of breastfeeding.

In 2007, the Centers for Disease Control and Prevention inaugurated the Maternity Care Practices Survey, which is designed to monitor maternity care practices that impact breastfeeding outcomes at all U.S. hospitals and birth centers. The CDC plans to continue assessing breastfeeding-related maternity care practices every other year, and to benchmark facilities against those of comparable size, as one way to encourage improvement in maternity care practices, and thus is breastfeeding outcomes.

In this book the reader will find many strategies to improve such practices gathered from the hospitals and birth centers from around the world that have pioneered the journey to improved practice as well as research that supports practice change.

Continuity of care is the delivery of health care over time, across settings, and across practices and disciplines, and is an ideal way to achieve the goal of patient-centered care. In Chapter One, we explore evidence-based policy as a cornerstone of continuity of care because we have come to understand that mothers experience continuity of care differently than do members of the healthcare system. For mothers, care is horizontal, meaning that they experience it as they move through time in the health system. So discrepancies in care over time are magnified when one person tells them one thing and another something else, even

if the first advice was appropriate for a baby of 1 day, and the second appropriate for a baby of 10 days old. The mother feels a lack of continuity. Because of this, it is imperative for us to work to achieve vertical continuity, that is, building agreement about breastfeeding and lactation management throughout the peripartum period.

In Chapter One we also explore the conundrum of breastfeeding as an art or a science and the impact of each worldview on continuity of care. Continuity of care is best achieved through agreement of evidence-based policy—which is not opinion in writing—and is best developed by an interdisciplinary team of equals. The chapter concludes with steps in policy development, the role of intuition, obstacles to evidence-based policies, and guidance on developing a breastfeeding policy for the maternity setting, including common barriers to the policy development process and strategies to overcome them.

In Chapter Two we explore the optimization of breastfeeding knowledge by assuring skill and competency throughout the health care system. We know from research studies that staff training can make a difference in breastfeeding outcomes, but policy and practice changes should be implemented in tandem with training. This chapter goes on to examine research relevant to the hallmarks of optimal training, what training should include, whether training should be mandatory, and adapting training to time and financial constraints.

Prenatal and perinatal teaching regarding infant feeding is the subject of Chapter Three. This chapter includes research about where prenatal breastfeeding education should best occur, expectations for breastfeeding education delivered in the healthcare system, evidence for the effect of prenatal breastfeeding education, common barriers to delivering prenatal breastfeeding education, and strategies for overcoming them.

The first hour after birth is critical to getting breastfeeding off to a good start, and medical routines are often at odds with biological needs during this period. We know about the dangers of separating newborn animals from their mothers, but we do not seem to understand the potential negative implications of separating human newborns from their mothers in the sensitive period immediately after birth. Chapter Four describes the expectations for the care of mothers delivering via vaginal and cesarean birth and their babies in the first hour as well as the evidence that supports keeping mothers and babies together during this critical time. We also discuss common barriers to optimal practice in the first hour of life, and strategies to overcome these barriers, such as routine procedures, education, and small scale research.

Beyond the first hour of life, breastfeeding assessment and support is needed. Chapter Five describes expectations for feeding evaluations, risk factors that decrease breastfeeding exclusivity and duration, as well as outcome measures for the postpartum period. The chapter goes on to explore the evidence for these interventions that appear in the research literature, as well as common barriers to optimal breastfeeding assessment and teaching, and strategies to overcome these barriers.

Healthy breastfeeding babies do not require routine supplementation with any food or drink other than breastmilk for the first six months of life. Chapter Six describes mecha-

nisms for assuring exclusive breastfeeding in the postpartum period. This chapter also includes a discussion of research related to the effect of supplementation on specific medical conditions as well as common nonmedical reasons for supplementation of the newborn. Contraindications to breastfeeding, as well as the effect of early supplementation on the baby, are included in this chapter as well. A discussion on supplementation requires examining the ethical and commercial problem of marketing formula to parents, and Chapter Six includes an exploration of this timely issue.

Optimal hospital and birth center policies and procedures promote rooming-in and eliminate routine nonmedical separations of mother and baby. There should be no routine delay between birth and the initiation of continuous rooming-in. Chapter Seven describes how to assure ongoing mother-baby contact by examining research supporting 24-hour rooming-in, as well as obstacles and solutions to achieving it.

Breastfeeding on demand has clear benefits compared with scheduled feedings, and has been described and recommended as the optimal breastfeeding strategy for many years. Chapter Eight examines the argument for breastfeeding on demand, the downside to encouraging restricted breastfeeding, and suggests strategies for teaching and assessment related to pacing the feedings. The chapter also includes strategies to overcome common barriers to implementation of unrestricted feeding.

In the early days of breastfeeding, the mother and baby are learning the intimate dance of feeding. During this time, it is best to avoid extracurricular suckling and feeding. Although pacifiers and bottles are sometimes considered synonymous with infancy, the general public is largely unaware of the negative impact these devices may have on breastfeeding. Chapter Nine presents policy expectations regarding the use of bottle nipples and pacifiers with healthy full-term breastfeeding infants, the evidence of the effects of exposure on breastfeeding outcomes, evidence related to other methods of supplementation, and suggestions for overcoming common barriers to reducing exposure to bottles and pacifiers.

The vast majority of a successful breastfeeding experience goes on outside the walls of the maternity facility; however, what happens during the maternity stay has a profound long-term effect on feeding outcomes including whether or not the staff provide linkage between the mother and breastfeeding resources outside the facility. Chapter Ten discusses mechanisms to bridge the gap between the maternity stay and the community, including policy expectations, evidence for the importance of on-going breastfeeding support, and common barriers to providing ongoing support and strategies to overcome these obstacles.

The WHO/UNICEF Baby-Friendly Hospital Initiative (BFHI) as a tool for change is the subject of Chapter Eleven. The BFHI is an international program that links breastfeeding with the health care themes of quality improvement, evidence-based practice, and family-centered care. As of 2008, there were approximately 20,000 Baby-Friendly designated hospitals and maternity centers throughout the world. The philosophic touchstones of the U.S. BFHI are objective, inclusive, accessible, voluntary, and celebratory, and these touchstones are discussed in Chapter Eleven. Chapter Eleven also includes a description of the journey toward Baby-Friendly designation for U.S. birth facilities, as well as the means used to evaluate the implementation of the Ten Steps to Successful Breastfeeding. The chapter concludes with the benefit of participation in the BFHI.

Chapter Twelve explores the qualitative aspects of breastfeeding care that have been found beneficial in assisting the mother and baby in attaining comfortable, effective, confident breastfeeding practices. The chapter asks and answers the question "What do we know about how women want to be helped by their caregivers?" by examining research evidence that leads us to understand a mother-based approach. Unfortunately, women are often silent about their needs and expectations, particularly in interchanges with systems such as health care settings. The chapter challenges us to discover the needs and wants of breastfeeding women by asking the true experts: the women themselves.

Practice change is the key to improving breastfeeding outcomes and quality improvement is a proven strategy for practice change. Chapter Thirteen suggests quality improvement tools and strategies that have been found useful to ascertain what information we have, defining the problem, differentiating the problem from what ought to be happening, and think about what the situation would look like without the problem.

Implementing best practice is a journey of change. Rarely is change easy. Nonetheless, we owe it to our clients—babies, mothers, and new families—to improve practices to foster the best possible outcomes. Our babies are our future!

Ten Steps to Successful Breastfeeding
A Joint WHO/UNICEF Statement[a]

Every facility providing maternity services and care for newborn infants should:

1. **Have a written breastfeeding policy that is routinely communicated to all healthcare staff.**
2. Train all healthcare staff in skills necessary to implement this policy.
3. Inform all pregnant women about the benefits and management of breastfeeding.
4. Help mothers initiate breastfeeding within a half-hour of birth. (US, one hour)
5. Show mothers how to breastfeed, and how to maintain lactation even if they should be separated from their infants.
6. Give newborn infants no food or drink other than breastmilk unless *medically* indicated.
7. Practice rooming in—allow mothers and infants to remain together—24 hours a day.
8. Encourage breastfeeding on demand.
9. Give no artificial teats (US, nipples) or pacifiers (also called dummies or soothers) to breastfeeding infants.
10. Foster the establishment of breastfeeding support groups and refer mothers to them on discharge from the hospital or clinic.

[a] World Health Organization. (1989). *Protecting, promoting and supporting breast-feeding: The special role of maternity services.* Geneva, Switzerland: World Health Organization, p. iv

CHAPTER

1

Evidence-Based Policy

A Cornerstone of Continuity of Care

No matter where we travel, mothers tell us the same thing—"I wanted to breastfeed but everyone in the hospital told me something different. I didn't know who to listen to, so I just gave up." This chapter is about how to help mothers by developing breastfeeding policies that are evidence based and foster continuity of care.

Developing policy really is the first, and most basic, step to implementing evidence-based continuity of care, but it can be a frustrating, politically charged, and drawn-out process. But, it is just that, a P-R-O-C-E-S-S. By working through the intricacies of policy, by working through the worries and issues raised by team members, you can establish a platform that will assure continuity of care.

In this chapter, we will discuss some of the barriers we have seen maternity care facilities face and overcome on their journey to optimal care for mothers and babies. Remember, getting there is half the fun.[b]

Continuity of Care = Quality, Seamless, and Coordinated Care

Continuity of care, the delivery of health care over time, across settings, and across practices and disciplines is an ideal way to assure seamless, coordinated, quality delivery and achieve the goal of patient-centered care (see Box 1-1).[1] Continuity of care spans interpersonal aspects of care (such as having a single primary care provider giving coordinated care) as well as the coordination of care throughout the healthcare system, among many institutions and providers.

Helping women breastfeed presents many challenges to continuity of care because there is an inherent time continuum extending throughout the childbearing years, encompassing primary care before and after conception, the peripartum and postpartum periods, as well as multiple specialties of primary care, obstetrics/gynecology, neonatol-

---

[b] The now unused slogan of the Cunard Cruise Line.

Box 1-1	**Patient-Centered Care**

Patient-centered care is "respectful of and responsive to individual patient preferences, needs, and values and ensuring that patient values guide all clinical decisions."

Source: Institute of Medicine. (2005). *Crossing the quality chasm: A new health system for the 21st century.* Washington, DC: National Academy Press, p. 6.

---

ogy, perinatology, and pediatrics. However, achieving continuity of care has been shown to be important to the mother's feelings and her relationship with the baby[2] and is associated with forming a personal and satisfying relationship between the mother and the health professional related to infant feeding communication.[3]

Freeman describes continuity of care as having three dimensions: *relational* continuity, *management* continuity and *informational* continuity.[4] Each of Freeman's three dimensions of continuity of care[5] applies to the care of the breastfeeding woman and her baby.

- *Relational continuity*—support and encouragement of the breastfeeding woman through the development of a trusting and satisfying relationship—should be assured through the establishment of a personal relationship with a care provider who has the knowledge and skill to facilitate the mother's infant feeding decisions.

- *Management continuity*—seamless care—should be assured horizontally (through time) and vertically (across disciplines). Seamless care for the breastfeeding mother and her baby presents special challenges because of the inherent segmentation of the healthcare system. The mother may have a different provider from her infant; she will probably have different nurses for every shift during her hospital stay, and the maternity nurses will be different from those who will care for her in the community. If specialized lactation care and services are available, they may be delivered only in the hospital, only on some days and shifts, or only in the community via mother-to-mother support and/or healthcare provider and/or a specialized lactation care giver, and rarely in both settings by the same provider throughout the breastfeeding experience.

- *Informational continuity*—Freeman's third dimension, assures that members of the healthcare team have access to medical records and test results pertinent to giving care. In the other direction, informational continuity assures that the mother is given consistent messages and teaching across settings and personnel. In a segmented healthcare delivery system, there are many challenges to informational continuity around breastfeeding. The mother may believe that there is informational continuity and assume that all of her care providers as well as the baby's are knowledgeable about every aspect of her history. For example, the mother may have a physical constraint to breastfeeding (such as being HIV positive) of which the baby's care provider is unaware, or she may think that the baby's provider knows that she has had breast reduction surgery when in actuality, the baby's provider in the community may have no access to the mother's health history.

Mothers experience care horizontally, through time, and are often heard to complain that every nurse in the hospital tells them something different about how to breastfeed and that their physicians tell them something different entirely. Such a mother is expressing frustration with the lack of *vertical* continuity of care (across disciplines), which she experiences *horizontally* (across time). See Box 1-2.

Nurses and physicians complain that another healthcare provider tells the mothers something that conflicts with their teaching. The lactation care provider may be marginalized because the information that she gives to mothers is different from that of the hospital staff. To achieve continuity of care for the breastfeeding mother and her baby, relational, management, and informational continuity must be assessed and addressed. This begins with understanding the various points of view related to breastfeeding.

Is Breastfeeding an Art or a Science?

Because *lactation* is a physiologic process while *breastfeeding* is a social process (see Box 1-3),[6] the words and concepts are not interchangeable. As a physiologic process, lactation and lactation management fit nicely into the healthcare setting. Medical, dietetics, and nursing school curricula include information about *lactation* (the physiological process) and if *breastfeeding* is addressed at all, it is from a problem-oriented point of view—sore nipples, mastitis, or slow weight gain.

The skills and techniques of breastfeeding, the social process, have been passed for millennia from one generation of women to another as a learned experience. Girls grew up watching their neighbors and female relatives breastfeed and listening to older, more experienced women solve breastfeeding problems. Sadly, because of several generations of women not breastfeeding at all or not breastfeeding in public, breastfeeding knowledge, techniques, and skills have become lost, muted, and distorted. Breastfeeding management knowledge from prior generations was situated largely in lay or folk knowledge and outside of the healthcare system.

Box 1-2   Mothers Experience Care Horizontally

Gerri decided to breastfeed even before she got pregnant. At 24, she was the first in her friendship group to have a baby. When asked how she knew that breastfeeding was right for her, she said, "I don't know. I've never even seen anyone breastfeed except in pictures and paintings; it just seems like the right thing to do." Although she never wavered from her desire to only breastfeed her baby for the first 6 months, Gerri received advertising mailings from formula companies beginning right after her first visit to the obstetrical practice. On the postpartum unit bottles of formula were placed on the baby's crib's shelves. Gerri had no problems with breastfeeding, yet when she was leaving the hospital the nurses gave her two bags of formula promotion materials and six extra bottles of ready-to-feed formula. When the baby was 2 weeks old, she received a coupon in the mail worth $5 off of a formula purchase.

She told her lactation care provider how difficult it was to receive all these formula samples. "I felt that no one was listening to me. I told them I wanted to breastfeed. In the hospital, I sent the first discharge bags back, but the next shift brought me more. My pediatric nurse practitioner offered me samples at the first well-baby check, even after I'd told her that I was planning to exclusively breastfeed for six months. When I went for my six week obstetric visit, the receptionist asked me if I'd like information about weaning or supplementing. I lost it! I started crying—what did they know that I didn't know? Was there some indicator that breastfeeding wouldn't work out for me and my baby? Were they listening to me at all?

The Moral of the Story: When the horizontal experience of the client is observed, we can see many ways in which the system was not honoring her plans, which were for optimal feeding! It is crucial to be aware of the confidence-eroding effects of this type of product promotion. No doubt the individual care providers involved thought they were doing something nice for the mother and baby by offering samples; however, the effect of these "gifts" can be devastating.

In recent decades, breastfeeding supporters and advocates have worked to reclaim this

Box 1-3   Lactation vs. Breastfeeding

"Whilst lactation is a physiological process, breastfeeding itself is a social behaviour, which has to be learned in an integrated, supportive system."

Source: Hauck, Y., Langton, D.,& Coyle, K. (2002). The path of determination: Exploring the lived experience of breastfeeding difficulties. *Breastfeeding Review;* 10(2), p 6.

social process through their personal experiences and observations of individual cases. Today, breastfeeding helpers may or may not have a healthcare background. They may or may not have had years of experience passively learning about breastfeeding through social interactions. They may approach the work of helping lactating women breastfeed as a science or as an art. Meanwhile, the irrefutable risks related to not breastfeeding, breastfeeding briefly, and mixed feeding have energized and engaged the medical and scientific community in promotion and support activities while defining breastfeeding through the more narrow lens of lactation. This results in health system expectations of brief medicalized contacts (see Box 1-4) to solve breastfeeding problems with prescriptive solutions (creams, pumps, gadgets) because social interactions are lengthy and anathema to the healthcare system.

The Challenge of Caring for a Dyad

The dual nature of the mother/baby dyad increases the challenge of continuity of care. While many care situations require careful coordination of care, childbearing, birth and breastfeeding add to that challenge by requiring that healthcare workers who typically focus on one aspect of care (maternal or pediatric) work together to support optimal outcomes for the mother and baby as a dyad who are dependent upon one another to make breastfeeding successful. Policy and procedure development teams must take this duality into account. What is done in the best interests of the mother must reconcile with the best interests of the baby, and vice versa.

Evidence-Based Practice—Where Does It Fit?

The intertwining of these two perspectives—lactation as a physiologic process (science) and breastfeeding as a social interaction (art) does not promote an optimal environment for interdisciplinary discussion and exploration of evidence-based policy development—the cornerstone of continuity of care. One extreme perspective values research and denigrates experience (science) and the other values experience over evidence (art). Further eroding the perceived value of science is the fact that healthcare workers and consumers are bombarded with questionable scientific research and information from a multitude of contradictory sources.

| Box 1-4 | If I Only Had the Time—The Visiting Nurse Dilemma |

Letty had been a rural visiting nurse for more than 10 years, changing dressings, organizing medications, and giving care to a largely geriatric population. When her employer decided to take on home visits to new mothers, she jumped for joy. Before going to work for the home visiting agency, Letty had worked in the hospital nursery, and, although she liked eldercare, she was excited to return to her first love, maternal-child health.

But she found the work frustrating because the agency expected her to spend the same amount of time with a new mother, a first-time breastfeeder, as she had with her other visits. "They simply don't understand that with new mothers you are seeing *two* people, the mother and the baby. They are only being reimbursed for the visit, so they expect me to do 6 or 7 or more visits in a day in a large rural area. I usually don't get to observe the baby breastfeeding or to thoroughly assess the mother for postpartum depression. I feel bad, really. These new mothers need more time, but the system just doesn't recognize these visits for how important and complex they are."

In the same news cycle, breast milk might be lauded as a way to decrease sudden infant death syndrome (SIDS), and hours later breast milk is under suspicion for containing harmful pollutants.

In addition, an ever-changing and expanding volume of research makes it impossible for clinicians to apply critical appraisal to each new bit of information. As a result, individual healthcare practitioners may be tempted to rely on nonevidence-based sources of information such as past practice, product promotions, or remembered training. Textbooks may not be reliable for answers to questions either, because by the time textbooks reach the shelves, new research is likely to have been published refuting some statements and adding new information. Efficient review, critical appraisal, and integration of new information and techniques are therefore crucial to providing optimal care across disciplines through evidence-based policies.

Objectively examining the validity of common health provider practices entails careful formulation of the presenting problem, evaluation of existing knowledge and research regarding treatment options, and integration of new information into evidenced-based policies. The issue increases in complexity when practitioners try to achieve continuity of care across disciplines and settings as is the case with the care of the breastfeeding mother and her baby.

The evidence-based practice paradigm can offer tools to address the tension between science and art, folklore and medicine, and between observed experience and authority by serving as the platform for policy development. The development of evidence-based policies, education regarding the implementation of the policy, and quality improvement oversight to assure optimal policy implementation are the strategies that integrate evidence-based practice and continuity of care.

The recent explosion in the publication of lactation research and systematic reviews, such as the meta-analysis, can be of great assistance to those seeking to develop evidence-based services for their settings. Evidence-based policy development provides a forum for interdisciplinary discussion, increasing knowledge of outcomes associated with common practice, and building consensus regarding best practices in breastfeeding care.

Policy Development—Not Opinion in Writing

Policy is best developed by an interdisciplinary team of equals. Although it is difficult, the team should allow scientific evidence, not the personalities and opinions of the team members, to guide the policy. The team should start out by making ground rules and agree to use a hierarchy of evidence such as the one that is described later in this chapter. One special problem that healthcare workers have in developing policy is an embedded belief in the healthcare system of autocratic rule, the idea that people with higher authority can make a decision alone and do not have to follow the rules of evidence—indeed do not have to follow the rules of logic even. This comes from a long autocratic tradition called *medicine by authority*.

Medicine by authority "rests on the assumption that the authority in question has comprehensive scientific knowledge. Understandably no one can."[7] Early societies believed that gods caused illnesses and since these higher authorities caused the illness, a higher authority would be needed to treat the illness. In the age of Descartes, physicians came to view the body as machinelike, capable of breaking, hence needy of formal tests and measurements and ultimately repair. This view challenged the premise that illness had godlike causes, yet the idea of authority remained.

The traditional paradigm of medicine by authority was based on the following four assumptions:[8]

1. *Authority is based on the amount of clinical experience a healthcare professional has had.* The foundation for diagnosis is built on one's own experience treating other patients. A clinician with 20 years of experience has more authority than a clinician with 2 years experience. We could think that breastfeeding helpers with years of experience, including breastfeeding their own children, would have the advantage in this assumption.

2. *Scientific foundation for practice is lodged in pathophysiology.* The body is understood as a complex machine; pathophysiology is the basis of the repair manual. Lactation management fits into this paradigm, but breastfeeding as a social process does not.

3. *Personal and clinical experience and/or collective judgment equip a practitioner to evaluate new ideas, tests, or procedures.* Published research studies are less important than one's own evaluation in this assumption. See Box 1-5 for an example.

4. *Mastery of subject areas (as in classroom experience) and clinical experience (as in residency, mentorships, and internships) are the prerequisites to clinical practice.* This assumption supports acquisition of breastfeeding and lactation knowledge in

---

Box 1-5   Using Personal Experience to Guide Practice

Dr. Nick had a reputation for encouraging breastfeeding, and his growing pediatric practice attracted many of the families in the community for whom breastfeeding the baby was a priority. Advocates in the community were puzzled that as supportive as Dr. Nick seemed to be about breastfeeding, he always recommended formula supplements to be given by bottle by the father every evening and overnight starting when the baby was a month old, even if the baby was growing well on only breast milk.

One day, at a hospital pediatric meeting, he told one of the residents his rationale. When his wife was breastfeeding their baby, who was a month old in the middle of December, she became exhausted by shopping and holiday preparations. Short-tempered, she was coping poorly with life in general. He began to help by feeding their baby formula in the evening and overnight. He thought it was such a good idea that he now advises every family to do the same.

Dr. Nick was not practicing patient-centered or evidence-based care. His recommendations were not based on either medical need or research, but rather on his own experience with his own child.

formal settings and acquiring credentials rather than acquisition of knowledge socially as in learning from breastfeeding mothers.

When practicing by authority, a clinician has a number of options, such as looking to personal experience (his or her own or family members' experience with breastfeeding), to what was learned in school about biology (which may not be supported by new research), looking up the problem in a textbook (which may be out of date), or asking an expert (who may or may not have helpful, evidence-based information).

Using Evidence to Guide Policy Development

Evidence-based practice is healthcare work based on scientific evidence rather than authority, clinical experience, or intuition alone. Employing evidence to guide policy development involves making thoughtful, reasoned decisions that integrate well-examined scientific evidence with clinical experience. In order to use evidence in this way, critical appraisal skills are needed. Access to information is also an integral part of making reasonable decisions based on critical appraisal. New information and scientific evidence concerning health becomes available every day. There is a constant need for updating and synthesizing knowledge.

According to Grimes,[9] the three assumptions of evidence-based practices are:

1. *Use outcome measures that have been evaluated and reproduced in a systematic manner.* Outcome measures can increase the certainty of diagnosis, treatment, and the validity of diagnostic tests.

U.S. outcome measures for breastfeeding, according to the Healthy People 2010 goals, include increasing the national breastfeeding initiation rate from the 1998 baseline of 64% to at least 75%, increasing the national rate of breastfeeding at 6 months from the 1998 baseline of 29% to at least 50%, and increasing the rate of breastfeeding for a least 1 year from 16% in 1998 to 25% in 2010. This requires closing a gap of 9%. In addition, exclusive (full) breastfeeding is expected, with goals at 40% for the proportion of mothers who exclusively breastfeed their infants at 3 months and 17% for the proportion who exclusively breastfeed at 6 months. Reaching these targets will require tightening of unnecessary supplementation in birth settings and the immediate postpartum, as only 50.9% of breastfed infants born in 2004 were receiving only breastmilk at 7 days of age.[10] Healthcare settings may also develop outcomes measures and quality improvement goals. These are discussed in Chapter 13.

2. *Pathophysiology is understood as only one part of knowledge.* Knowledge of outcome measures, risks, interpersonal skills, spiritual life, and community support are also important.

This is especially crucial in developing breastfeeding policies, because the social process is the other part. In addition, pathophysiology knowledge related to lactation has changed dramatically in the past few years. New understanding of the milk-making and delivery structures inside the breast, for example, give us radically different insight into lactation than was known even 2 years ago.

3. *Formal rules of evidence,* raised later in this chapter, are used to evaluate the literature.

Traditionally, the medical sector focused on healers who provided care for individuals when they were sick, while the population-oriented public health sector focused on promoting healthful conditions for the community at large. The emphasis of medicine, then, was on healing individual illness and the emphasis of public health was on population-based disease prevention. Over time, and with no economic incentives for the two sectors to collaborate, separate and independent health systems developed in the United States. The two health sectors compete for the limited resource of healthcare dollars.

Changes in the healthcare system in recent decades, restructured according to the rules of the marketplace, and the redefinition of the government's role in public health, have created an environment of growing interdependence between medicine and public health. Breastfeeding is an obvious example of the public health sector's findings of positive health outcomes associated with breastfeeding pushing back onto the healthcare delivery system. The problem is compounded when breastfeeding is promoted in the public health sector and maternity care practices provide suboptimal support.

The First Steps in Policy Development

The policy development group (committee or team) should be composed of a workable number of staff members, usually a number between five and twelve. It's optimal to have representatives from all of the affected departments and disciplines, with an amiable, respected coordinator. The chair/coordinator need not be a breastfeeding expert. In many cases, the group is more productive if the chair/coordinator has had policy-writing and/or group facilitation experience, and staff members with breastfeeding or lactation expertise serve the group as technical consultants.

Developing a policy is an educational and interactive process, and because of this, reluctant and unconvinced staff members may become more committed to supporting breastfeeding during the course of the policy development work. Anyone pulling a policy team together should consider including skeptical staff members on the policy team for this reason.

When writing a breastfeeding policy, the team should begin with critical appraisal. The self-appraisal tool from UNICEF/WHO[11] is a good place to start the appraisal. This is a detailed process, with several steps described next:

- Precisely define the problem through careful interviewing, history taking, and observational skills. For example, the group might want to achieve 24-hour rooming in in the hospital for at least 80% of the mothers and babies. First, the team has to know what the current situation is. What percent of mothers are currently rooming in for 24 hours? Why and when are babies in the nursery except for medical reasons? What do the mothers say when they ask that their baby be removed to the nursery? Is there a difference between the use of the nursery by women who have had vaginal births compared to women who have had cesarean births?

The team should consider a patient survey that would help them to understand what the mother's experience was like. In one survey,[12] 75% of mothers who had breastfed at the first feeding had problems with breastfeeding, yet only 25% of these mothers reported that they received help for their problem during the hospital stay.

- Determine what is needed in order to solve the problem (see Box 1-6 for a sample situation).

- Conduct an efficient and thorough literature search, perhaps using an online search engine such as PubMed,[13] which comes from the U.S. National Library of Medicine (NLM) and National Institutes of Health (NIH). Develop a list of keywords, print out all of the abstracts, and get full copies of all of the pertinent articles to review in their entirety.

- Select the studies that are relevant to the problem. This means those with the best research, not the studies that agree with a preconceived hunch.

- Extract the clinical message from the research.

- Apply the message to the problem.

What are the best research studies to guide clinical practice? What published information should be considered as evidence when developing a policy? Each article should be examined in relation to its validity and applicability. Critical appraisal "comprises the ability to assess the validity and applicability of clinical, paraclinical, and published evidence and to incorporate the results of this assessment into clinical management."[14]

An excellent resource for evidence-based policy development is the classic series of articles written by Greenhalgh[15] on the theme how to read a paper, published in the *British Medical Journal*. Another resource is the series of articles "User's Guides to the Medical Literature," written by Guyatt, Sackett, Sinclair, Hayward, Cook, and R. J. Cook[16]

Box 1-6 **What Is Needed in Order to Solve the Problem?**

Faraday Hospital was working to implement the *Ten Steps to Successful Breastfeeding,* but when it began its critical appraisal of its Level 1 nursery usage, it found that babies were spending hours each morning in the nursery waiting for their pediatric exams and waiting for transport back to their mothers' rooms. All of the babies on the unit were collected between 7 and 7:30 a.m. while their mothers were showering and eating breakfast, and they remained in the nursery after their pediatric exams until the nurses had a chance to bring them back to their mothers' postpartum rooms. A stumbling block was that the pediatricians were resistant to changing the practice, citing that exams would be impossible to do accurately in the postpartum rooms because of poor lighting. The hospital installed improved lighting in the postpartum rooms so that the babies could be examined without transporting them to the nursery.

and published in the *Journal of the American Medical Association.*

The Hierarchy of Evidence

There are several ways to weigh one study against another. We like the process that Guyatt and colleagues[17] published a hierarchy of evidence, weighing research from most reliable to least reliable. See Table 1-1.

It is also important for a policy development team to be able to identify the relative level of inherent bias in the research the members are reading, as well as asking themselves questions in order to extract the message and apply it to the case at hand.

There are benefits and disadvantages of all study designs. For example, while randomized, controlled trials can allow rigorous examination of a single treatment variable, they are expensive to conduct and therefore more likely to be sponsored by commercial interests or to have a small sample size. The evidence hierarchy can provide perspective on the merits of various study designs and findings. Studies can also have problems and conditions that need to be taken into consideration. Loss of participants, a different population than the policy team's, or other issues with the study may make it less relevant. What the policy team should not do

Table 1-1	**Hierarchy of Evidence**
Research Design	**Definition**
Systematic reviews and meta-analyses	Systematic review is an overview of primary studies using explicit, reproducible methods.
	Meta-analysis is a mathematical synthesis of results of two or more primary studies.
Randomized, controlled trials	Participants are randomly allocated to treatment or control groups. Randomized, controlled trials with definitive results are ranked more highly than those with nondefinitive results.
Cohort studies	Two or more groups of people are selected on the basis of difference in their exposure to a potentially causal agent, and outcome is followed.
Case-controlled studies	Subjects with a certain condition are paired with control subjects matched for other factors; data is collected and outcomes observed.
Cross-sectional surveys	A representative sample of subjects are interviewed or studied. Data is collected to gain answers to specific clinical questions.
Case reports	Anecdotal reports of specific experiences of individuals are collected.

Greenhalgh, T. (1997). How to read a paper: Papers that summarize other papers (systematic reviews and meta-analyses). *British Medical Journal 315*: 672.

Greenhalgh, T. (1997). How to read a paper: Getting your bearing (deciding what the paper is about). *British Medical Journal 315*:243.

Source: Based on Guyatt, G. H., Sackett, D. L., Sinclair, J. C., Hayward, R., Cook, D. J., & Cook, R. J. (1995). User's guides to the medical literature. IX. A method for grading health care recommendations. *Journal of the American Medical Association, 274*, 1800–1804.

is to find a study that supports a particular point of view and reject all of the others that do not. Although this technique can be very tempting, is not evidence based.

Is There a Role for Intuition or Experience in Policy Development?

The use of intuition or experience in policy development poses a challenge to the evidence-based paradigm. Intuition can be an important guide to questioning and developing hypotheses; however, it must be used with caution. It is important for policy developers to examine intuitive thoughts and feelings carefully, as they have the potential to be both illuminating and misleading.

When developing breastfeeding policy, team members may find it helpful to use intuition and experience in guiding the process of interviewing staff members and consumers, as well as when defining and hypothesizing the problem. However, it is important to stop and reflect on the problem in the process of writing policy. After hypothesizing, the team members should think critically about not only the information in hand but also about the information that is missing. They mustn't write anything into the policy without solid evidence, no matter how strong the force of intuition or experience.

Many, if not all, clinicians and breastfeeding specialists are prone to developing personal attachments to certain policies and procedures. These attachments can form thought filters that block admission of new information, especially if it conflicts with the favored way of giving care. Read Box 1-7 for an example of thought filtering. The challenge to clinicians and breastfeeding specialists is to develop breastfeeding policies that foster continuity of care through integrating critical appraisal and fostering openness to new information.

Box 1-7   **Discovering Thought Filters to Policy Implementation**

The policy development team at a community hospital was working to improve breastfeeding outcomes by reducing the amount of formula supplementation given to breastfed babies without medical indication of need in the first 24 hours. The critical appraisal process led the team to believe that the first hour after birth was key. If the baby could be allowed to stay uninterrupted, skin to skin with its mother, until self-attaching to the breast, the team was convinced that that later breastfeeding would be more successful.

When the team presented their ideas to the delivery staff, many obstacles were raised. The biggest problem was that current policy required the baby to be admitted to the nursery, necessitating transport away from the mother. In addition, the delivering physician or midwife was required to record the baby's weight prior to leaving the facility. The weighing and admission process became thought filters in the policy development process. Once these barriers were uncovered, new policies that addressed them could be developed.

Obstacles to Evidence-Based Policies

Grimes[18] describes five obstacles to implementing healthcare practice based on evidence. We have applied each of these potential obstacles to evidence-based breastfeeding policies:

1. *Seduction by Authority:* This is the absorption of tenets of breastfeeding authorities as truth—writing nonevidence-based practices into policy on an expert's say-so, often proceeded by "I heard such and such expert say at a conference..."

2. *False Idol of Technology:* This is a situation that involves allowing commercial interests to shape policy. "If we buy it, it must be good. Let's write a policy around it." This is how policy becomes undermined by technology. For example, newborn babies placed in warming cots stay *colder* for longer than they do with skin-to-skin holding.[19] Yet, in many hospitals, babies have to be placed on warmers until they reach a certain temperature rather than spending that time warming up faster on their mothers' chests.

3. *Let Sleeping Dogmas Lie:* These are unexamined assumptions that certain techniques and products work ("this is the way we've always done it") so they are not even brought forth for policy consideration. For example, a policy that says that hypoglycemic babies must be fed one ounce of formula and does not mention expressed colostrum or breastfeeding for breastfed babies contains the unexamined (and untrue) presumption that formula is quickly available and of known caloric value while colostrum or mother's milk is neither available nor suitable.

4. *Pursuit of Pedantry:* This happens when there is a lack of dialogue with other disciplines (for example, not engaging the marketing department in the discussion about replacing formula discharge bags with hospital logo bags) and nomenclature skirmishes (e.g., clutch vs. football hold; let-down vs. milk ejection; formula vs. artificial baby milk; etc.).

5. *Numerators in Search of Denominators:* This is the rejection or distortion of research messages in the interest of protecting current beliefs and practices of the field. For example, a policy that discourages smoking mothers from breastfeeding because of an image of only "pure" mothers breastfeeding, when feeding formula and exposing the baby to second-hand smoke is the worst choice for the baby.

Many products and techniques in current usage have never been studied adequately to examine their safety and efficacy. Some products have not even been studied prior to manufacture by the producer! Breast shells and exercises that have been advertised and recommended for decades for use in the treatment of inverted nipples are one example. After a large randomized, controlled trial[20] of these devices, researchers found that sustained improvement was most likely in the nontreated control group. Women who were assigned to use the product (breast shells) were the least likely to be successful at breastfeeding and their nipples were no more likely to evert than those of women with similar nipples who did nothing to prepare them.

It is strongly recommended that practitioners seek out and develop an evidence base for all interventions. Beliefs such as "It's natural; it can't hurt;" "Ancient people did it this way—it must be OK;" or "This gadget is being sold for this problem. It will help" must be viewed with the same skeptical eye as thalidomide, diethylstilbestrol (DES), and routine episiotomy. Well-conducted, unbiased outcome evaluation is the best available tool to determine the safety and efficacy of products and treatments.

Developing a Breastfeeding Policy for the Maternity Setting

Iker and Mogan[21] found that continuing education (of nurses) alone did not assure compliance with a breastfeeding policy. They concluded that for a breastfeeding policy to be effective appropriate practices must be included, there must be a mechanism for monitoring staff practice, and outcome measurements should be monitored. Statements in support of breastfeeding have been issued by professional associations and are available to policy developers. These professional policies can be the starting point in developing institutional policies.

State a Purpose for the Policy Development Group

Working out the purpose of the group and writing it down helps everyone to know the parameters of the work. Here's an example:

To assure that the institution has a written, evidence-based policy that promotes continuity of care related to breastfeeding and delineates standards of care for breastfeeding mothers and babies.

Expectations for Breastfeeding Policy

Grizzard, Bartick, Nikolov, Griffin, and Lee[22] surveyed postpartum nurse managers at 43 (88%) maternity hospitals in Massachusetts to determine the degree of implementation of the policies of the WHO/UNICEF document, *Ten Steps to Successful Breastfeeding*, the first step of which is to "maintain a written breastfeeding policy that is routinely communicated to all healthcare staff."[23] Only 2% of hospitals were considered by the researchers to have a high implementation of the *Ten Steps to Successful Breastfeeding*. However, 58% were rated as having a moderately high level of implementation, 40% had a partial level, and none were implementing the 10 steps at a low level. Hospitals that accepted free formula were the most likely to have a negative association with overall implementation of the *Ten Steps to Successful Breastfeeding*.

What are the expectations of an institution related to a breastfeeding policy? At a minimum, the policy should be inclusive of the *Ten Steps to Successful Breastfeeding* and should have explicit directions for how the policy is to be routinely communicated to all healthcare staff. Also, the policy should be available so that the staff caring for mothers and babies can refer to it. The policy should have clear objectives and a means for determining, by audit, whether or not the policy is being practiced. There is more about this aspect of policy in Chapter 13.

The policy should be dated, and there should be a review cycle stated within the policy. Commitment to policy implementation is a requirement at every level of the facility, from the highest level of management to the lowest paid staff member who will be responsible for the quality of the policy in practice.

In addition, support for breastfeeding mothers and a summary of the policy should be posted in the areas of the facility that serve pregnant women, mothers, infants, and/or children in the languages used by the community.

■ Common Barriers to the Policy Development Process and Strategies to Overcome Them

The first barrier to policy development process that is often encountered when a breastfeeding policy is suggested is *resistance*. A common argument might be, "Why should there be a special policy on breastfeeding? We mention breastfeeding in our other policies." Our response is that it's only when breastfeeding policies and practices are laid out horizontally (across time) and vertically (across disciplines) that we are able to assure continuity of care. Many teams have found that it was only once they extracted all of the policies about breastfeeding or that would affect breastfeeding from all other facility policies that they could clearly see the conflicts and inconsistencies.

Looking at the horizontal experience of the mother and the baby gives insight into many common problems around separation and education. Looking at the vertical (across disciplines) policies and practices helps the team understand why there may be disagreements about care. Unwritten policies must be addressed. For example, the obstetrical care providers may be telling mothers not to breastfeed at night so they can rest and pediatric care providers are telling mothers that the baby must be fed during the night to assure adequate intake. Neither of these is expressed as a formal written policy, yet the nurses deal with the conflict on a daily basis. Looking at horizontal and vertical aspects of care will bring this kind of issue to light. At first, the policy team must remember that it is only doing a critical appraisal—getting the lay of the land. There is no need to *fix* the problem(s), only to identify the problem and its characteristics.

Individual staff members may express concern that focusing on breastfeeding will *make formula-feeding families feel guilty*. Breastfeeding is clearly the infant feeding method of preference vis-à-vis maternal and child health. However, there are situations in which formula is the appropriate feeding method, such as the infant or mother with a contraindicated condition (see the short list of these contraindications in Chapter 6, Box 6-2) and for infants of mothers who choose not to breastfeed. The impetus behind the 10 Steps is to provide informed decision-making and support optimal outcomes by improving maternity care practices. Mothers who do not wish to breastfeed should be supported in learning how to formula feed safely, once staff have ascertained that these mothers have received adequate education and counseling to have arrived at an informed decision. Prenatal education, routine skin-to-skin contact, education and counseling regarding feeding cues and mechanics, routine rooming-in, and referral to postpartum resources are expectations for the care of all families, not only those who have selected breastfeeding. Discussions around guilt should be reoriented to a discussion of improving practices to benefit all families.

Another barrier may be *lack of support from key sectors* (e.g., administrative, managerial, medical, nursing, etc.) to create a forum for discussing and revising policy. Breastfeeding may not be considered important enough or interesting enough compared to other health-care issues that confront the institution. If this is the case, the breastfeeding advocates should search out a *champion* among the hospital administration or management who can take on the leadership of the policy development. A mistake that is commonly made is to think that the person taking the lead must be passionate about breastfeeding mothers and their babies. A tepid champion is still a champion, and the process of working through the policy may stoke the flames of support. The breastfeeding policy development team should be multidisciplinary and include representatives of all key sectors. One hospital's breastfeeding team started small but grew by the month. By the time the Baby-Friendly assessors were ready to make an on-site visit, the committee had over 40 members. Its secret? A monthly newsletter that reached a larger group than those attending the meetings.

Because healthcare costs are always a concern, the *potential costs of policy change* may be a perceived barrier. Sweeping changes require reeducation of staff. Achieving an ethical business relationship with formula suppliers may mean that some of the benefits to the hospital are threatened. The money that a hospital saves the entire health system by improving breastfeeding outcomes is not rendered back to the hospital, so if a hospital increases its exclusive breastfeeding rate, the hospital does not directly benefit; the insurance companies who pay for fewer ear infections, gastrointestinal problems, and lower respiratory tract infections are the financial beneficiaries.

The team should present information regarding economic benefits of breastfeeding and the costs of artificial feeding to provide documentation of the benefits of breastfeeding and of the influence of maternity care practices on breastfeeding outcomes. In addition, it should get an unbiased appraisal of the cost of change to the institution and its calculated costs to determine the community benefits of improving breastfeeding outcomes.[24,25]

Another significant barrier is *putting policy into practice*. Translating policy into practice and knowledge into behavior is a challenge (see Box 1-8). This will be addressed in the chapters that follow, but the policy should specify monitoring or audit parameters that will be implemented to assure compliance.

Developing a breastfeeding policy is an enormous undertaking. The development team shouldn't minimize the importance of this work or the time it will take. The members should keep in mind that this is a *process*—a journey; they must try to hold onto a sense of humor. Changing policy and practice takes time. See the wise words of Sally Tedstone in Box 1-9.

Resource

The Academy of Breastfeeding Medicine Protocol Committee. (2007). ABM Clinical Protocol #7: Model Breastfeeding Policy. *Breastfeeding Medicine,*2(1), 50–55. Accessible at http://www.bfmed.org/index.asp?menuID=139&firstlevelmenuID=139.

References

1. Gulliford, M., Naithani, S., & Morgan, M. (2006). What is 'continuity of care'? *Journal of Health Services Research and Policy,* 11(4), 248–250.
2. Ekstrom, A., Widstrom, A. M., & Nissen, E. (2003). Breastfeeding support from partners and

---

"Although knowledge about the benefits of breastfeeding appear to have been well disseminated to mothers and to healthcare professionals, the translation of that knowledge into behavior lags behind."

Source: Lawson, M. (1998). Recent trends in infant nutrition. *Nutrition, 14,* 755.

Box 1-9 **The Process of Sustainable Change**

Infant Feeding Coordinator Sally Tedstone, R. M., A. D. M., Cert Ed. (F. E.) of St. Michael's Hospital in Bristol, United Kingdom, sums up the reality of sustainable change:

"Looking back, I think it was my experience of implementing Baby Friendly in another setting that had taught me that you cannot implement change successfully and sustainably by simply telling people what to do. You have to bring them along with you so that they understand why it is the right thing to do, and only effective education will do that."

grandmothers: Perceptions of Swedish women. *Birth, 30*(4), 261–266.

3. Hoddinott, P., & Pill, R. (2000, December). A qualitative study of women's views about how health professionals communicate about infant feeding. *Health Expectations, 3*(4), 224–233.

4. Freeman, G. K., Olesen, F., & Hjortdahl, P. (2003). Continuity of care: An essential element of modern general practice? *Family Practice, 20,* 623–627.

5. Freeman, G. K., Olesen, F., & Hjortdahl, P. (2003). Continuity of care: An essential element of modern general practice? *Family Practice, 20,* 624.

6. Hauck, Y., Langton, D., & Coyle, K. (2002). The path of determination: Exploring the lived experience of breastfeeding difficulties. *Breastfeeding Review, 10*(2), 5–12.

7. Grimes, D. A. (1995). Introducing evidence-based medicine into a department of obstetrics and gynecology. *Obstetrics and Gynecology, 86*(3), 451–457.

8. Grimes, D. A. (1995). Introducing evidence-based medicine into a department of obstetrics and gynecology. *Obstetrics and Gynecology, 86*(3), 452.

9. Grimes, D. A. (1995). Introducing evidence-based medicine into a department of obstetrics and gynecology. *Obstetrics and Gynecology, 86*(3), 452.

10. Centers for Disease Control & Prevention (2007) Table 3: Any and exclusive breastfeeding rates by age among children born in 2004. Retrieved from http://www.cdc.gov/breastfeeding/data/NIS_data/2004/age.htm on 02/11/08.

11. UNICEF/World Health Organization. (2006). Baby-friendly hospital initiative: revised, updated and expanded for integrated care. Retrieved from http://who.int/nutrition/topics/BFHI_Revised_Section_4.pdf on 12/15/07.

12. Baydar, N., McCann, M., Williams, R., Vesper, E. , & McKinney, P. (1997, November). Final Report: WIC Infant Feeding Practices Study. Washington, D.C.: United States Department of Agriculture, Food and Nutrition Service, Office of Analysis and Evaluation. Contract No. 53–3198–3-003.

13. May be accessed at http://www.pubmed.gov

14. Bennett, K. J., Sackett, D. L., Haynes, R. B., Neufeld, V. R., Tugwell, P., & Roberts, R. (1987). A controlled trial of teaching critical appraisal of the clinical literature to medical students. *Journal of the American Medical Association, 257*(11), 2451.

15. Greenhalgh, T. (1997). How to read a paper: Getting your bearing (deciding what the paper is about). *British Medical Journal, 315,* 243.

16. Guyatt, G. H., Sackett, D. L., Sinclair, J. C., Hayward, R., Cook, D. J., & Cook, R. J. (1995, December). Users' guides to the medical literature. IX. A method for grading health care recommendations. *Journal of the American Medical Association, 274*(22), 1800–1804.

17. Guyatt et al. Users' guides to the medical literature. IX. A method for grading health care recommendations.

18. Grimes, D. A. (1986). How can we translate good science into good perinatal care? *Birth, 13,* 2.

19. Christensson, K., Siles, C., Moreno, L. Balaustequi, A., De La Fuente, P., Lagercrantz, H., et al. (1992). Temperature, metabolic adaptation and crying in healthy full-term newborns cared for skin-to-skin or in a cot. *Acta Pediatr, 81*(6–7), 488–493.

20. Alexander, J. M., Grant, A. M., & Campbell, M. J. (1992). Randomized controlled trial of breast shells & Hoffman's exercises for inverted and non-protractile nipples. *British Medical Journal, 304*(6833), 1030–1032.

21. Iker, C. E, & Mogan, J. (1992, September). Supplementation of breastfed infants: Does continuing education for nurses make a difference? *Journal of Human Lactation, 8*(3), 131–135.

22. Grizzard, T. A., Bartick, M., Nikolov, M., Griffin, B. A., & Lee, K. G. (2006, May). Policies and practices related to breastfeeding in Massachusetts: Hospital implementation of the ten steps to successful breastfeeding. *Maternal Child Health Journal, 10* (3), 247–263.

23. World Health Organization. (1989). *Protecting, promoting and supporting breast-feeding: The special role of maternity services.* Geneva, Switzerland: World Health Organization, p. iv.

24. Ball, T. M., & Wright, A. L. (1999, April). Health care costs of formula-feeding in the first year of life. *Pediatrics, 103*(4 Pt. 2), 870–876.

25. Weimer, J. (2001, March). Food assistance and nutrition research report No. FANRR13. Retrieved from www.ers.usda.gov/Publications/FANRR13/ on 12/15/07.

Ten Steps to Successful Breastfeeding
A Joint WHO/UNICEF Statement[a]

Every facility providing maternity services and care for newborn infants should:

1. Have a written breastfeeding policy that is routinely communicated to all healthcare staff.
2. **Train all healthcare staff in skills necessary to implement this policy.**
3. Inform all pregnant women about the benefits and management of breastfeeding.
4. Help mothers initiate breastfeeding within a half-hour of birth. (US, one hour)
5. Show mothers how to breastfeed, and how to maintain lactation even if they should be separated from their infants.
6. Give newborn infants no food or drink other than breastmilk unless *medically* indicated.
7. Practice rooming in—allow mothers and infants to remain together—24 hours a day.
8. Encourage breastfeeding on demand.
9. Give no artificial teats (US, nipples) or pacifiers (also called dummies or soothers) to breastfeeding infants.
10. Foster the establishment of breastfeeding support groups and refer mothers to them on discharge from the hospital or clinic.

[a] World Health Organization. (1989). *Protecting, promoting and supporting breast-feeding: The special role of maternity services.* Geneva, Switzerland: World Health Organization, p. iv

CHAPTER 2

Optimizing Breastfeeding Knowledge, Skill, and Competency Throughout the Healthcare System

■ The Importance of Having Skills for Providing Breastfeeding Care

Every provider who cares for mothers and babies should have the knowledge and skills necessary to provide quality breastfeeding care. As we visit maternity care facilities around the world, we have observed two ways of thinking about breastfeeding knowledge and skill. In the first, all maternal-child staff members are competent and engaged in helping breastfeeding mothers and babies. In the other, breastfeeding competency is concentrated in a few designated staff members. Spreading the responsibility for breastfeeding care throughout the facility's staff assures that needed services will be available vertically and horizontally. In our experience, facilities that concentrate competence, knowledge, and skill meet overwhelming obstacles in providing continuity of breastfeeding care. In this model, the breastfeeding caregiver spends the majority of their work time helping mothers and babies to overcome obstacles to breastfeeding created by care practices that do not favor optimal breastfeeding.

Although breastfeeding initiation rates climbed in the 1970s from just over 20% to more than 50% by 1982, breastfeeding was considered a *lifestyle* choice for women in the United States. By and large, the medical community was at best indifferent, at worst discouraging, to breastfeeding. Women who breastfed past the early weeks were sometimes told they were doing it for themselves since human milk was thought to have little value. The thinking was that the new formulas had been manufactured scientifically and were superior to the old evaporated milk and homemade concoctions. These formulas were thought to surpass human milk in nutrition and convenience, making breastfeeding obsolete.

One reason that breastfeeding wasn't thought to make any difference in either the mother's or the baby's health in industrialized nations was that much of the published medical research supporting the concept of breastfeeding as a *public health priority* was conducted in parts of the world where

breastfeeding was shown to decrease the rates of acute illness and death of babies and young children. With few U.S. babies dying from diarrhea and pneumonia, research from other parts of the world didn't resonate among healthcare providers. It wasn't until research indicated that exclusive and long-term breastfeeding might decrease the risk of high-cost chronic conditions, such as obesity, cancer, and diabetes, that it also began to be considered a *public health issue* in the United States and some other industrialized countries. In the spring of 2007, the federal agency for Healthcare Research and Quality (AHRQ) published its review of research related to the advantages and disadvantages of breastfeeding in developed countries and laid to rest the concern that there may not be actual benefits to breastfeeding outside of developing countries. Prior to this report, the argument was always made that the health of breastfed babies and their mothers in developed country settings was due to the availability of clean water, adequate healthcare, etc.[1]

During the time when breastfeeding was considered only a lifestyle issue, there was no need to include substantive theoretical or practical knowledge about breastfeeding management in the curriculum of physicians, nurses, dieticians, or other healthcare providers. Lactation, the physiologic production of milk, might be included, but breastfeeding, the social process, was not. Even healthcare providers who had chosen to specialize in the area of maternal and child health—obstetricians, pediatricians, pediatric nurse practitioners, and maternal child health nurse specialists—might have had very little lactation or breastfeeding education included in their preservice curriculum; they gave advice based on their own experience and whatever limited information about lactation they had received in their education.

Research studies investigating the knowledge and attitudes of health professionals regarding breastfeeding have been published. Attitudes, practices, and recommendations by obstetricians about infant feeding were studied in one county in New York. The physicians who were surveyed reported that their training in infant feeding was inadequate.[2] Pediatricians in training were found to have "extremely limited knowledge of breastfeeding management" in a California study.[3] A national random survey of pediatric residents and pediatricians, who were board certified within the previous 3 to 5 years, indicated that residency training "does not adequately prepare pediatricians for their role in breastfeeding promotion."[4]

An earlier study[5] found that despite the recommendations of the Academy of Pediatrics, almost one half of the pediatricians surveyed did not routinely recommend breastfeeding. Family practice residents and practicing physicians were surveyed to determine whether they had received adequate training and education about breastfeeding to promote and manage breastfeeding among their patients. The researchers found that many respondents were not only unaware of the many advantages of breastfeeding, but they also scored low on clinical management knowledge.[6] A questionnaire was distributed to family practice residents in Georgia and North Carolina. Sixty-seven percent of residents stated that their training in breastfeeding counseling was inadequate.[7]

Barnett, Sienkiewicz, & Roholt, found that "although most health professionals had positive beliefs about breastfeeding, differences by profession, work environment, and personal breastfeeding experience indicate the need for comprehensive training in lactation management."[8] Freed, Clark, Sorenson, Lohr, Cefalo, and Curtis investigated the adequacy of breastfeeding knowledge of residents and practicing physicians in pediatrics, obstetrics/gynecology, and family medicine and found that "physicians were ill prepared to counsel breast-feeding mothers." They concluded "deliberate efforts must be made to incorporate clinically based breast-feeding training into residency programs and continuing education workshops."[9]

Bagwell, Kendric, Stitt, and Leeper studied the breastfeeding knowledge and attitudes of dietitians, nurses, and physicians in Alabama.[10] They found that dietitians expressed stronger interest in breastfeeding and exhibited greater knowledge of questions asked than nurses. Attitude and knowledge scores of physicians were not statistically different than those of dietitians and nurses. In a study of dietitians, physicians, and nurses in Utah hospitals, Helm, Windham, and Wyse found that dietitians were the least likely to provide breastfeeding information and assistance.[11] The authors conclude: "standard nursing and dietetics training programs have failed to include sufficient education and training to give either of these professionals the proper skills to manage lactation. Nurses, as well as dietitians, must seek out additional education on their own."[12]

Lewinski examined the knowledge base of a sample of obstetrical nurses at three different maternity hospitals.[13] Nurses in the study populations completed a survey of 16 questions testing their knowledge regarding breastfeeding. Only 7 of the 16 questions were answered correctly by more than 50% of the respondents. The authors conclude that "staff nurses working in OB units continue to teach mothers outdated information related to breastfeeding."[14]

One way of judging educational curriculum is to examine the textbooks used in pre-service education of healthcare professionals to determine whether or not they contain comprehensive, accurate, or up-to-date information. Philipp and Merewood[15] concluded that the breastfeeding information in pediatric textbooks that they examined as part of a research study was highly variable and, at times, inconsistent and inaccurate. Using a standardized scoring sheet, they examined eight U.S. texts published between 1999 and 2002. Three reviewers evaluated each book for inclusion of 15 basic predetermined breastfeeding topics and found that the mean number of basic breastfeeding topics identified in each text was 11; accurate, up-to-date information was lacking in many.

A common base of knowledge and skills is desirable both to achieve the breastfeeding objectives and—equally important—to support the ongoing development, evaluation, and modification of breastfeeding policies through evidence-based practice and data-driven planning. The challenge is to provide members of this diverse provider group with opportunities for training, education, and credentialing that will address breastfeeding issues while promoting personal career development objectives. Although almost all national and international statements regarding breastfeeding and human lactation call for changes to improve education for healthcare providers and lactation manage-

ment based on evidence, changing current practice is a slow process that needs a well thought-out plan.

Not everyone who cares for mothers and babies has to be knowledgeable at the same depth. Naylor, Creer, Woodward-Lopez, and Dixon[16] have suggested three levels of complexity, or depth, for lactation management education. See Box 2-1.

The healthcare provider's own perception of his or her knowledge may not be a good indication of actual knowledge, according to research conducted by Becker,[17] who reported about a survey of health professionals' knowledge conducted in three rural maternity units in Ireland. According to survey results, the unit where breastfeeding rates had increased the most in 3 years had the highest scores, the greatest number of staff with maximum scores, and the only professional with a postgraduate qualification in breastfeeding. Staff in the other units (where rates had fallen or risen only slightly) felt that they had enough knowledge about breastfeeding to assist mothers. Their main source of information was infant formula manufacturers through regular visits of company representatives, study events on infant feeding supported by formula manufacturing companies, and printed information that formula manufacturing companies provided for mothers.

■ Staff Training Makes a Difference in Breastfeeding Outcomes

We know from research studies that staff training can make a difference in breastfeeding out-

---

Box 2-1   **Breastfeeding Education/Complexity**

Level I: Awareness

Target group: medical students (preservice education).

Example objective: Describe the general benefits of breastfeeding for the infant.

Level II: Generalist

Target group: pediatricians, obstetric-gynecology physicians and residents, family medicine residents, and advanced practice nurses.

Example objectives: Apply the findings from the basic and social sciences to breastfeeding and lactation issues.

Describe the unique properties of human milk for human infants.

Describe the advantages of preterm milk for preterm infants.

Level III: Specialist

Target group: those in advanced/independent study, fellowships.

Example objective: Critique the findings from the basic and social sciences and evaluate their applicability to clinical management issues.

Discuss in detail the components of human milk and their functions.

Describe in detail the suitability of preterm human milk for preterm infants.

Source: Naylor, A. J., Creer, A. E., Woodward-Lopez, G., & Dixon, S. (1994). Lactation management education for physicians. *Seminars in Perinatology, 18,* 525–531.

---

comes, but *policy and practice changes should be implemented in tandem with training.* Winikoff and Baer[18] examined research studies in an early systematic review of the literature in order to understand which medical practices promoted optimal breastfeeding outcomes. They reported that education without policy and practice change did not significantly change breastfeeding outcome. One of the least influential practices was education of healthcare providers alone, without policy change, hence the recommendation that education should include clinical skills and the construction of policy that supports best practice.

Hallmarks of optimal training include that it is *specific to the staff competencies necessary for the implementation of a breastfeeding policy.* In a 2004 study by Cantrill, Creedy, and Cooke,[19]

for example, although midwives understood the importance of early skin-to-skin contact between the mother and baby, continuous uninterrupted skin-to-skin contact was not understood and rarely practiced.

In a study of the knowledge and practice outcomes from a 3-day course, Valdes, Pugin, Labbok, Perez, Catalan, Aravena, et al. .[20] reported changes in the clinical breastfeeding support practices of 100 health professionals in Chile. Included as course topics were clinical skills and policy considerations related to the physiology of lactation, lactational infertility, and breastfeeding management strategies. The authors concluded that this didactic and participative course improved participants' knowledge and practices. Similar findings by other researchers including Davies-Adetugbo and Adebawa,[21] who studied breastfeeding outcomes of mothers who were seen by community health workers in rural Nigeria, indicate that courses that combine theoretical knowledge and practical skills may improve breastfeeding outcomes by improving workers' knowledge and practices.

Several research studies have examined breastfeeding outcomes as a measure of training success. For example, Taddei, Westphal, Venancio, Bogus, and Souza[22] and Cattaneo and Buzzetti[23] found that a training course on breastfeeding practices that increased the knowledge of healthcare workers could affect breastfeeding outcomes. In the case of Taddei et al., exclusive breastfeeding increased by 29% and full breastfeeding increased by 20%. Cattaneo et al. report that the knowledge scores of health professionals increased from 0.41 to 0.72 in one group of hospital staff and from 0.53 to 0.75 in the other after taking the 3-day course. The rates of exclusive breastfeeding at discharge improved from 41% to 77% in mothers from the first group of hospitals where staff were trained and from 23% to 73% in the second group. The rates of full breastfeeding and any breastfeeding at 3 and 6 months postpartum also improved.

Hillenbrand and Larsen[24] measured the impact on knowledge and confidence related to breastfeeding of an interactive multimedia curriculum. They studied 49 pediatric residents in the United States by measuring knowledge and confidence and resident behaviors before and after the training. Mean knowledge scores increased from 69% before to 80% after the training. Mothers reported receiving breastfeeding-appropriate clinical practices 22% of the time prior to training and 69% after the training.

Vittoz, Labarere, and Castell[25] also looked at the increase in breastfeeding duration as a result of an intensive 3-day training program for maternity ward professionals who worked with healthy term babies in a French university hospital. The result of the before-and-after study with 2 retrospective random samples of 308 mothers indicates that a 3-day training program can increase the duration of breastfeeding, in this case from 13 weeks breastfeeding to 16 weeks.

■ What Should the Training Include?

WHO and UNICEF have offered a 20-hour course to support the Baby-Friendly Hospital Initiative (see Box 2-2) and have developed objectives, curriculum, and knowledge checks[b] (see Box 2-3) specific to the field of breastfeeding and human lactation for staff members of hospitals working to implement the *Ten Steps to Successful Breastfeeding*. All staff with primary responsibility for the care of breastfeeding mothers and babies should have a minimum of 20 hours of training.

As shown in the studies reported previously, this training often occurs over 3 days and includes *didactic* as well as *practical* and *counseling approaches* to helping mothers breastfeed.

Training should include practical clinical experience because classroom teaching can be insufficient or irrelevant to work practice. In

---

[b] Each section is a separate file and may be downloaded from UNICEF at http://www.unicef.org/nutrition/index_24850.html, or by searching the UNICEF web site: http://www.unicef.org or the WHO web site: www.who.int/nutrition.

Box 2-2	**The UNICEF/WHO 20-Hour Course**

Breastfeeding Promotion and Support in a Baby-Friendly Hospital: A 20-Hour Course for Maternity Staff

According to UNICEF and the World Health Organization:

The 20 hours may be presented in three intensive days or in shorter segments over a longer period, whichever is most suitable for the facility. It is intended that every hospital staff member who has direct patient care responsibility for mothers and babies will attend the course. It is kept short in anticipation that it will need to be repeated within the same hospital in order to reach all staff from all shifts.

A 20-hour syllabus allows much of the essential information to be presented. There are 15.5 hours of classroom time focused on skill-oriented training including discussion and pair practice. The 4.5 hours of clinical practice provides time with pregnant women and new mothers inclusive of 3 or more hours of competency verification. Training for other staff members may be tailored to their job description and degree of exposure to breastfeeding.

Source: UNICEF/World Health Organization. (2006). *Baby-Friendly Hospital Initiative: Revised, updated and expanded for integrated care.* Retrieved October 18, 2007, from: http://www.who.int/nutrition/topics/BFHI_Revised_Section_3.1.pdf.

Box 2-3	**Knowledge Checks from the UNICEF/WHO 20-Hour Course**

Breastfeeding Promotion and Support in a Baby-Friendly Hospital: A 20-Hour Course for Maternity Staff

A colleague asks you why this course is taking place and how it would help mothers and babies that you care for. How will you reply?

List two reasons why exclusive breastfeeding is important for the child.

List two reasons why breastfeeding is important for the mother.

What information do you need to discuss with a woman during her pregnancy that will help her to feed her baby?

List two antenatal practices that are helpful to breastfeeding and two practices that might be harmful.

If a woman is tested and found to be HIV positive, where can she get infant feeding counseling?

/continues

Box 2-3	**Knowledge Checks from the UNICEF/WHO 20-Hour Course**

Breastfeeding Promotion and Support in a Baby-Friendly Hospital: A 20-Hour Course for Maternity Staff (continued)

Mark the answer T (True) or F (False).

1. Giving mothers company-produced leaflets about breast milk substitutes can affect infant feeding practices.   T   F
2. Breast milk substitutes include formula, teas, and juices (as well as other products).   T   F
3. The International Code and BFHI prohibit the use of formula for infants in maternity wards.   T   F
4. Health workers can be given any publication or materials by companies as long as they do not share these publications with mothers.   T   F
5. Donations of formula should be given to mothers of infants in emergency situations.   T   F

List four labor or birth practices that can help the mother and baby get a good start with breastfeeding.

List three ways to assist a mother following a cesarean section with breastfeeding.

Name three possible barriers to early skin-to-skin contact and how each might be overcome.

Explain how you would describe to a new mother how to tell if her baby is well attached and suckling effectively.

What are the four key points to look for with regard to the baby's position?
Suppose you are watching Donella breastfeed her 4-day-old baby. What will you look for to indicate that the baby is suckling well?

Give three reasons why rooming-in is recommended as routine practice.

Explain as you would to a mother what is meant by demand feeding or baby-led feeding.

List three difficulties or risks that can result from supplement use.

Keiko tells you that she thinks she does not have enough milk. What is the first thing you will say to her? What will you ask her in order to learn if she truly does have a low milk supply?

You decide that Ratna's baby, Meena, is not taking sufficient breast milk for his needs. What things can you do to help Ratna increase the amount of breast milk that her baby receives?

/continues

| **Box 2-3** | **Knowledge Checks from the UNICEF/WHO 20-Hour Course** |

Breastfeeding Promotion and Support in a Baby-Friendly Hospital: A 20-Hour Course for Maternity Staff (continued)

Jacqueline has a 33-week preterm baby in the special care nursery. It is very important that her baby receive her breast milk. How will you help Jacqueline get her milk started? How will you help her with putting the baby to her breast after a few days?

Yoko gives birth to twin girls. She fears she cannot make enough milk to feed two babies and that she will need to give formula. What is the first thing you can say to Yoko to help give her confidence? What will you suggest for helping Yoko breastfeed her babies?

List four reasons why it is recommended that mothers learn to hand express.

List four reasons why cup feeding is preferred to feeding by other means if the baby cannot breastfeed.

What breastfeeding difficulties would suggest to you that you need to examine a mother's breasts and nipples?

Rosalia tells you she became painfully engorged when she breastfed her last baby. She is afraid it will happen with the next baby, too. What will you tell her about preventing engorgement?

Bola complains that her nipples are very sore. When you watch her breastfeed, what will you look for? What can you do to help her?

Describe the difference between a blocked duct, noninfective mastitis, and infective mastitis. What is the most important treatment for all of these conditions?

A pregnant woman says to you that she cannot breastfeed because she would need to buy special foods for herself that she could not afford. What can you say to her to help her see that breastfeeding is possible for her?

A coworker says to you that a mother will need to stop breastfeeding because she needs to take a medication. What can you reply to this coworker?

List three sources of support for mothers in your community.

Give two reasons why mother-to-mother support may be useful to mothers.

/continues

Box 2-3 **Knowledge Checks from the UNICEF/WHO 20-Hour Course**
Breastfeeding Promotion and Support in a Baby-Friendly Hospital:
A 20-Hour Course for Maternity Staff (continued)

Give two reasons why breastfeeding is important to the older baby and the mother.
List two reasons why a hospital might seek BFHI external assessment.

Explain, as if to a coworker, why achieving Baby-Friendly designation is not the end of the process, and explain the importance of ongoing monitoring.

Source: UNICEF/World Health Organization. (2006). *Baby-Friendly Hospital Initiative: Revised, updated and expanded for integrated care.* Retrieved October 18, 2007, from: http://www.who.int/nutrition/topics/BFHI_Revised_Section_3.1.pdf

---

2003, Cantrill, Creedy, and Cooke[26] examined how Australian midwives learned about breastfeeding and found that on-the-job experience was the most valuable learning activity cited by the more than 1000 survey respondents. Only 3.1% of respondents rated their hospital or university education program as a valuable breastfeeding information source. Sloper, McKean, and Baum[27] found that there is no change in outcome unless there is a practical component to the training. Training should provide competency verification in the practice setting in order to assure that learning has taken place. Minimal competencies are listed in Box 2-4. Readers should not make the mistake of substituting technology for skill (see Box 2-5).

Training should also be directed toward changing attitudes, especially attitudes that create barriers to competent care. Some health workers have negative attitudes towards breastfeeding, which may be strengthened by negative personal experience with breastfeeding (see Box 2-6). Ekström, Widstrom, and Nissen[28] provide an approach, process-oriented training, that

may assist in helping staff with negative attitudes. Their research was conducted with antenatal midwives and postnatal nurses in Sweden. Ten antenatal and child health centers were randomized to intervention and control groups. The intervention training offered participants an opportunity to explore attitudes and knowledge in a supportive environment. Attitudes measured included regulating, facilitating, disempowering, and breastfeeding antipathy. One year after the training, the midwives in the intervention group were found to have lower scores on breastfeeding antipathy. The postnatal nurses' scores decreased on regulating and disempowering scales and increased on facilitating breastfeeding. The authors conclude that the process-oriented training improved the participants' attitudes towards breastfeeding and decreased their need to schedule and control maternal breastfeeding behavior.

Sometimes, the training can change a staff member's attitude because after the training they now feel capable and competent. Staff resistance to assisting breastfeeding mothers

---

Box 2-4   **Competency Requirements**

Each maternity care setting will have its own set of staff competencies required to assure optimal breastfeeding outcomes for mothers and babies, but at a minimum staff should be able to:

- Counsel mothers about infant feeding choices with the understanding that although breastfeeding is optimal, the choice is ultimately the mother's to make.
- Assist the mother with skin-to-skin care immediately after birth and throughout the postpartum stay.
- Accurately assess the breastfeeding baby's latch-on and suckling for potential or current problems.
- Teach the nursing mother how to breastfeed and how to maintain lactation if separated from her baby.

- Teach the mother how to hand express her milk.
- Cup feed a baby safely.
- Teach parents how to feed by cup if appropriate and necessary.
- Teach the mother how to recognize feeding cues and respond to them by feeding the baby.
- Counsel the mother regarding pacifier use.
- Counsel the mother regarding the use of bottles and formula.
- Provide evidence-based answers to parents' common questions and concerns regarding breastfeeding.
- Refer the mother to sources of appropriate postpartum breastfeeding support.

Box 2-5   **The Slippery Slope of Substituting Technology for Skill**

A colleague told us about her experience tabulating the results from an infant feeding study.

We interviewed 100 first-time mothers who had given birth at five different hospitals about their birthing and breastfeeding experiences. As we reviewed the interviews we saw a pattern with the 29 mothers who had all delivered at the same hospital. Almost every one had problems with beginning breastfeeding, especially with latching their babies on. Every mother went home pumping and feeding their baby away from the breast, leaving it to community

breastfeeding supporters and the visiting nurses to assist the mother toward her goal of breastfeeding (Anonymous).

The Moral of the Story: Technology (such as pumps, nipple shields, and other tools) may be overused when staff lacks the skill to help mothers and babies. One way to determine staff competency and training needs is to monitor the use of breastfeeding gadgets such as breast pumps and nipple shields. The use of formula without medical indication is also a good indicator of level of staff skill and competency.

Box 2-6   The Power of Processing Personal History

Jennifer is a 50-year-old nurse with more than 20 years of experience in the obstetrics setting. As a young nurse, she came to love supporting breastfeeding women and looked forward to breastfeeding her own children. However, when her first baby was born, she had a very difficult time with breastfeeding. Her nipples were truly inverted. She asked for help from her colleagues, but none were able to help her, and many told her to just tough it out. She had difficulty getting her firstborn son to latch on, and started pumping and bottle-feeding her milk to her son. Juggling pumping and feeding her pumped milk became more difficult. After about 2 weeks, her milk supply dwindled, and she gave up attempting to collect her milk. Her nipples were very sore, and she had bruising and trauma to her areolae from trying to evert her truly inverted nipples. She felt very sad about the loss of the breastfeeding experience she had always dreamed of, and didn't even attempt to breastfeed her other children. She attempted to share these feelings with her coworkers, her partner, her friends, and her family, but her feelings were dismissed by all. She was told, "You should be happy you have a healthy baby," and "He got your milk for a couple of weeks—that's all he needed." No one offered to simply listen as Jennifer processed her feelings or empathized with the loss of this experience she had so eagerly anticipated.

Jennifer felt that she had failed as a mother, and that the medical system had failed to support her. As a result, she came to be quite brusque with her patients who told her they wanted to breastfeed. "It's really going to hurt," she would tell them. "You've got to be tough." In her opinion, she was helping prepare these women for the reality that they would be on their own, without support, if they chose to try breastfeeding. Essentially, she was trying to protect her patients from her own experience.

When her hospital mandated breastfeeding training for the staff, Jennifer strongly resisted attending. She didn't want to have to encounter those feelings again. Finally her manager told her that not attending the program would have negative ramifications on her annual salary review, and Jennifer grudgingly agreed to be scheduled for the training program. During the sessions, she was quite vocal about breastfeeding being painful and less important than the instructor was saying it was. She argued that all the videos and pictures shown were of women with perfect nipples, stating that anyone could help those women breastfeed. After the second class, the instructor asked Jennifer to go out for a cup of coffee with her. Surprised, Jennifer agreed. As they sat over coffee, the instructor said in a kind voice, "You have lots of strong feelings about breastfeeding. Can you tell me what has led you to think it's so difficult?" The floodgates opened. Jennifer revealed her story of pain and loss, and was shocked by how much emotion was locked up in that experience, even though her son was now 24 years old! The instructor offered lots of empathy and listened to Jennifer until she ran out of words. She then said, "I can certainly see why you feel so strongly about breastfeeding. I am so sorry that you didn't receive the support you needed. What a terrible loss that was for you! I would like to encourage you to think about how your own experience affects the work you do now. Would you be willing to have coffee with me again after the next class? Here is my phone

/continues

| Box 2-6 | **The Power of Processing Personal History (continued)** |

number—please call me anytime if you'd like to discuss this further."

The Moral of the Story: Some health professionals who have had children have not had happy breastfeeding experiences. Others may have unresolved feelings about receiving inappropriate or inadequate information or support. These experiences and feelings can stand in the way of delivering quality care. It is crucial that trainers, supervisors, and coworkers offer to process personal history. Helping caregivers to process personal experiences can be an important step to putting them aside so that these experiences no longer color the support offered to new families.

can reside in feelings of lack of competence or confidence. Thus, a clear focus of training must be to assure competence and confidence in the ability of staff members to assist mothers and babies with breastfeeding.

Staff training should be mandatory. Iker and Mogan[29] found that when training was voluntary, outcomes and practice did not change. In Box 2-7 you can read about Paula's experiences offering staff training at the hospital in which she worked.

The World Health Organization/UNICEF Baby-Friendly Hospital Initiative (BFHI) curriculum recommends at least 20 hours of training, including at least 4.5 hours of clinical practice. This is a recent increase from the original 18-hour course because new topics have been added based on 15 years of international experience with the initiative. Short-duration training has not been demonstrated to change attitudes. Martens[30] reports on the effectiveness of a 1.5-hour mandatory training session for all nursing staff in a rural Canadian hospital. This session was designed to increase exclusive breastfeeding, create positive breastfeeding beliefs and attitudes,

and increase compliance with the 10 steps. Outcomes at this hospital were compared with those at a control site before and after the intervention. Seven months after the training, increases were seen at the intervention site on compliance with the 10 steps, breastfeeding knowledge, and exclusive breastfeeding rates (31% prior, 54% after), but no change occurred in breastfeeding attitudes.

Longer training sessions are also effective. The UNICEF/WHO 40-hour breastfeeding counseling training course[31] has been shown to be effective in improving skills of health workers. In a study by Rea, Venancio, Martines, and Savage,[32] 60 health professionals (one per health facility) were randomly allocated to an intervention group ($n=20$) who attended the course, or a control group ($n=40$). Qualitative and quantitative methods were used to evaluate the impact on participants' breastfeeding knowledge, skills, and attitudes immediately after the course (early posttest) and 3 months later (late posttest). Indicators measuring knowledge, clinical skills, and counseling skills showed a significant increase in the intervention

---

Box 2-7   Don't Save the Worst for Last

Paula faced an uphill battle in improving breastfeeding services at the hospital where she worked. As a registered nurse and lactation consultant, Paula had been a staff member for more than 20 years as the institution went from one administration and one crisis to another. Obstetrics (OB) nurse managers came and went, sometimes only staying for a few weeks, while the nursing staff averaged 22 years tenure. The situation had resulted in postpartum/OB/nursery nurses who were tired of change and believed that the need to help mothers with breastfeeding was just another new trend to be endured. If they waited long enough, they thought, Paula would just give up and go away.

Optimistically, Paula organized a course around the *Ten Steps to Successful Breastfeeding*, received permission from the current administrator and nurse manager to pay staff for attendance hours, and signed up volunteers for her first class. She received an enthusiastic response and the class was fully subscribed in a matter of hours. The response to Paula's teaching was gratifyingly enthusiastic. Paula organized a second class on the heels of the first.

It took longer to fill the second class and Paula felt some resistance while teaching.

> There seemed to be some hostility with the second group. I thought at the time that I had a couple of gripers and complainers, but I figured once they got back to their units and joined in with the nurses who had taken the first class, they would see that I wasn't kidding about how much nicer it would be for them if they knew the reasons behind the breastfeeding initiative and knew how

> to help mothers. I started doubting my ability to teach during this class series. I felt as though some of the nurses were throwing up every barrier they could to try to defeat me. I was so grateful for the nurses in the class who got it and supported me. I was so happy when that class series was over!

When Paula looked at the list of who was left to take the class after the first two series she was stunned.

> As I looked at the list I realized what has happened and how I went wrong. By letting people sign up for the classes I got most of the enthusiastic, supportive nurses in the first class series, with only a few in the second. They were the ones I got help from in the second group. Now, the only ones who were left were the real problem nurses. The ones that are the most negative, the angriest, the ones least likely to change. I couldn't bear to even imagine what the classes would be like. I gave up.

The Moral of the Story: Find another way to organize your class participation other than volunteering. You might end up facing a nightmare class at the end, without a single supporter in the room. Paula's advice:

> I realize now that nurses who support breastfeeding will always be the first to sign up for anything that has "breastfeeding" in the title. If I had to do it over again, I would do it in alphabetical order, zip code, birthday months … anything but volunteers.

group in the early posttest, which decreased only slightly in the late posttest. The biggest change was observed in the counseling skills: listening and learning, nonverbal communication, and building confidence and giving support.

Refresher training may be needed to sustain improvements in breastfeeding outcomes, according to research by Prasad and Costello.[33] Before the 10-day training program, breastfeeding was initiated within 24 hours of birth by 29% of the preintervention mothers. Immediately following the training, breastfeeding initiation improved to 84%. However, 6 months after the training, only 59% of mothers had started breastfeeding within 24 hours of birth. This helps us understand the need to audit outcomes and refresh skills and competencies.

Common Barriers to Implementing Staff Training & Strategies for Overcoming Them

The training modality should be adapted to *time and money constraints.* Plans to train staff about breastfeeding policies and procedures may stall when questions arise about how to accomplish a mammoth job on a miniscule budget with little time. All staff who have daily contact with mothers and babies should be trained, and traditionally we think of training taking place in groups and located in a classroom for hours at a time. In addition, staff turnover, the need for updates, and reinforcement all add to the cost.

In many settings, the cost of training includes paying the trainer and buying materials, paying staff for the time they are in class *and* paying for other workers to provide patient care. When one adds up all the numbers, it's easy to see how training can become a significant barrier to improving breastfeeding outcomes!

To cut down on costs, first, one should *assess prior education* offered through in-service sessions, skills labs, conferences, etc. to determine where content needs have already been provided. The minimal competency checklist (Box 2-5) can be used to determine which skills are being practiced optimally and which are not. For example, one may find that although some staff attended a workshop that included the advantages of breastfeeding, staff don't seem to translate their learning into counseling. Mothers complain, and one observes that staff badger pregnant women and use judgmental language when talking about breastfeeding. In this case, the training plan should focus on counseling skills, rather than on learning the reasons to breastfeed.

Thinking out of the box addresses both time and money questions. Those planning a training session should consider the following:

- Think in terms of spreadsheets instead of attendance lists. Think about objectives, knowledge modules, and competencies and base the spreadsheets on these.

- Examine the possibility that training can take place during staff meetings and during staff downtime when there is low patient census. Learning can take place in small increments if the curriculum is planned to accommodate the reality of the setting.

- In-house training may be more or less expensive compared to imported expertise.

The in-house trainer may find it helpful to attend a train-the-trainer class. Check the resource list at the end of the chapter for ideas.

- Maternity care facilities have used self-study training modules acquired from outside vendors. The resource list at the end of the chapter will help you get started.

- Consider web-based training. The resource list at the end of the chapter will help you get started.

- Construct learning modules from recent journal articles and quiz questions that the trainer constructs. Choose articles that address the issues in the 20-hour course. Be sure that the training plan addresses the knowledge checks (Box 2-3).

Updating staff training is an arduous task, but a necessary one. Training should be targeted to assisting staff in making practice changes. Most professionals need to know *why* they should change practice, not just *what* should change.

Resources

AWHONN. (1998). *Achieving consistent quality care.* Washington, DC: Association of Women's Health, Obstetric and Neonatal Nurses.

Best Start Social Marketing. (2001). *Health care provider kit.* Tampa, FL: Author.

Breastfeeding Support Consultants. (1995). *Creating change . . . in the face of resistance.* Chalfont, PA: Breastfeeding Support Consultants

Cadwell, A. L., & Turner-Maffei, C. (1999). *Toward evidence-based breastfeeding practice.* Sandwich, MA: Health Education Associates, Inc.

Cadwell, K. (1997). Using the quality improvement process to affect breastfeeding protocols in United States hospitals. *Journal of Human Lactation, 13,* 5–9.

Cadwell, K. (Ed.). (2006). *The curriculum in support of the Ten Steps to Successful Breastfeeding: An 18 hour interdisciplinary breastfeeding management course for the United States.* Washington, DC: US Department of Health and Human Services. This curriculum and supporting educational media is available from Health Education Associates. The Healthy Children Project offers a train-the-trainer course to accompany this curriculum.

Cadwell, K., & Turner-Maffei, C. (Eds.). (2002). *Ten Steps to Successful Breastfeeding.* Sudbury, MA: Jones & Bartlett Publishers. Accessible at http://Tensteps.jbpub.com.

Cattaneo, A., & Buzzetti, R. (2001). Effect on rates of breast feeding of training for the baby friendly hospital initiative. *BMJ, 323*(7325), 1358–1362.

Canadian Task Force on the Periodic Health Examination. (1979). The periodic health examination. *Canadian Medical Association Journal, 121,* 1193–1254.

DeGeorges, K. M. (1999). Evidence! Show me the evidence! Untangling the web of evidence-based health care. *AWHONN Lifelines, 3,* 47–48.

Dickersin, K., Manheimer, E. (1998). The Cochrane collaboration: Evaluation of health care and services using systematic reviews of the results of randomized controlled trials. *Clinical Obstetrics and Gynecology, 41,* 315–331.

Dolan, M. S. (1998). Interpretation of the literature. *Clinical Obstetrics and Gynecologyg, 41,* 307–314.

Enkin, M., Keirse, M. J. N. C., Renfrew, M., & Neilson, J. (1995). *A guide to effective care in pregnancy and childbirth* (2nd ed.). Oxford, England: Oxford University Press.

Family and Reproductive Health, Division of Child Health and Development. (1998). *Evidence for the Ten Steps to Successful Breastfeeding.* Geneva, Switzerland: World Health Organization.

Feldman-Winter, L., Mulford, C., & Touger-Decker, R. (2000). *Lactation for clinicians* [CD-ROM and web components]. Newark, NJ: University of Medicine and Dentistry of New Jersey. Available at http://www.umdnj.edu/lactweb/index.htm

Greenhalgh, T. *How to read a paper: The basics of evidence based medicine.* London: BMJ Publishing Group.

Guyatt, G. H., Sackett, D. L., Sinclair, J. C., Hayward, R., Cook, D. J., & Cook, R. J. J. (1995). User's guides to the medical literature. IX. A method for grading health care recommendations. *Journal of the American Medical Association, 274,* 1800–1804.

Health e-Learning.(n.d.) *Breastfeeding Essentials.* Queensland, Australia: Health e-Learning. Accessible at http://www.health-e-learning.com/content/blogcategory/16/77/.

Heinig, M. J. (1999). Evidence-based practice: Art versus science? *Journal of Human Lactation, 15,* 183–184.

International Lactation Consultant Association. (1999, April). Evidence-based guidelines for breastfeeding management during the first fourteen days. Raleigh, NC: International Lactation Consultant Association. [Revised as *Guidelines for the Establishment of Exclusive Breastfeeding,* 2005].

Kitson, A., Harvey, G., & McCormack, B. (1998). Enabling the implementation of evidence-based practice: A conceptual framework. *Quality in Health Care, 7,* 149–158.

Leff, E. W., Schriefer, J., Hagan, J. F., & DeMarco, P. A. (1995). Improving breastfeeding support: A community health improvement project. *The Joint Commission Journal on Quality Improvement, 21,* 521–529.

Livingstone, V. (2003). *On-Line Educational Program on Clinical Breastfeeding Management.* Vancouver, BC, Canada: University of British Columbia. Accessible at http://www.breastfeedingclinic.com/bfdvd/.

McKibbon, K. A. (1999). Evidence-based practice. *Bulletin of the Medical Library Association, 86,* 396–401.

O'Connor, M., & Lewin L. (1998). *Breastfeeding Basics.* Cleveland, Ohio: Case Western Reserve University. Accessible at http://breastfeedingbasics.org.

Sikorski, J., Renfrew, M. J. Pindoria, S., & Wade, A. (2002) Support for breastfeeding mothers. *Cochrane Database of Systemic Reviews,* (1):CD001141.

Simpson, K. R., & Knox, G. E. (1999). Strategies for developing an evidence-based approach to perinatal care. *Maternal Child Nursing, 24,* 122–131.

Sinclair, J. C., Bracken, M. B., Horbar, J. D., Soll, R. F. (1997). Introduction to neonatal systematic reviews. *Pediatrics, 100,* 892–895.

UNICEF. (1999). *Breastfeeding: Foundation for a healthy future.* New York: UNICEF.

UNICEF & World Health Organization. (2006). Baby-Friendly Hospital Initiative revised, updated and expanded for integrated care. Available at:\ http://www.who.int/nutrition/topics/BFHI_Revised_Section_3.1.pdf. Section 3.2 session outlines breastfeeding promotion and support in a baby-friendly hospital, a 20-hour course for maternity staff.

U.S. Preventive Services Task Force. (2003). *Breastfeeding counseling.* Washington, DC: U.S. Department of Health and Human Services.

Walker, M. (2006). *Breastfeeding management for the clinician: Using the evidence.* Sudbury, MA: Jones and Bartlett Publishers.

Wellstart International. (2004). *Lactation management self-study modules, Level I.* San Diego, CA: Author.

WHO. (2003). *Global strategy on infant and young child feeding.* Geneva, Switzerland: Author.

Wood, M. J. (2006). Nursing practice research and evidence-based practice. *Clinical Nursing Research, 15*(2), 83–85.

World Health Organization and Wellstart International. (1993). *Promoting breast-feeding in health facilities: A short course for administrators and policy makers.* Geneva, Switzerland: World Health Organization, WHO/NHD/96.3).

References

1. AHRQ. (2007, April). Evidence report number 153. Retrieved from: http://www.ahrq.gov/downloads/pub/evidence/pdf/brfout/brfout.pdf on 10/31/07.

2. Howard, C. R., Schaffer, S. J., & Lawrence, R. A. (1997). Attitudes, practices, and recommendations by obstetricians about infant feeding. *Birth, 24*(4), 240–246.

3. Williams, E. L. & Hammer, L. D. (1995). Breastfeeding attitudes and knowledge of pediatricians-in-training. *American Journal of Preventive Medicine, 11,* 26–33.

4. Freed, G. L., Clark, S. J., Lohr, J. A., & Sorenson, J. R. (1995). Pediatrician involvement in breastfeeding promotion: A national study of residents and practitioners. *Pediatrics, 96,* 490–494.

5. Michelman, D. F., Faden, R. R., & Gielen, A. C. (1990). Pediatricians and breastfeeding promotion: attitudes, beliefs and practices. *American Journal of Health Promotion, 4,* 181–186.

6. Schwartz, K. (1995). Breastfeeding education among family physicians. *Journal of Family Practice, 40*(3), 297–298.

7. Goldstein, A. O., & Freed, G. L. (1993). Breastfeeding counseling practices of family practice residents. *Family Medicine, 25,* 524–529.

8. Barnett, E., Sienkiewicz, M., & Roholt, S. (1995). Beliefs about breastfeeding: A statewide survey of health professionals. *Birth, 22*(1), 15–20.

9. Freed, G. L., Clark, S. J., Sorenson, J., Lohr, J. A., Cefalo, R., & Curtis, P. (1995). National assessment of physicians' breast-feeding knowledge, attitudes, training and experience. *Journal of the American Medical Association, 273,* 472–476.

10. Bagwell, J. E., Kendrick, O. W., Stitt, K. R, & Leeper, J. D. (1993). Knowledge and attitudes toward breast-feeding: Differences among dietitians,

nurses and physicians working with WIC clients. *Journal of the American Dietetic Association, 93*(7), 801–804.

11. Helm, A., Windham, C. T., & Wyse, B.. (1997). Dietitians in breastfeeding management: An untapped resource in the hospital. *Journal of Human Lactation, 13*(3), 221–225.

12. Helm, A., Windham, C. T., & Wyse, B.. (1997). Dietitians in breastfeeding management: An untapped resource in the hospital. *Journal of Human Lactation, 13*(3), 224.

13. Lewinski, C. A. (1992). Nurses' knowledge of breastfeeding in a clinical setting. *Journal of Human Lactation, 8*(3), 143–148.

14. Lewinski, C. A. (1992). Nurses' knowledge of breastfeeding in a clinical setting. *Journal of Human Lactation, 8*(3), 147.

15. Philipp, B. L., & Merewood, A. (2004). The baby-friendly way: The best breastfeeding start. *Pediatric Clinics of North America, 51*, 761–783.

16. Naylor, A. J., Creer, A. E., Woodward-Lopez, G., & Dixon, S. (1994). Lactation management education for physicians. *Seminars in Perinatology, 18*, 525–531.

17. Becker, G. E. (1992). Breastfeeding knowledge of hospital staff in rural maternity units in Ireland. *Journal of Human Lactation, 8*(3), 137–142.

18. Winikoff, B., & Baer, E. C. (1980). The obstetrician's opportunity: Translating "breast is best" from theory to practice. *American Journal of Obstetrics & Gynecology, 138*(1), 105–117.

19. Cantrill, R., Creedy, D., & Cooke, M. (2004). Midwives' knowledge of newborn feeding ability and reported practice managing the first breastfeed. *Breastfeeding Review, 12*(1), 25–33.

20. Valdes, V., Pugin, E., Labbok, M. H., Perez, A., Catalan, S., Aravena, R., et al. (1995). The effects on professional practices of a three-day course on breastfeeding. *Journal of Human Lactation, 11*(3), 185–190.

21. Davies-Adetugbo, A. A., & Adebawa, H. A. (1997). The Ife South Breastfeeding Project: Training community health extension workers to promote and manage breastfeeding in rural communities. *Bulletin of the World Health Organization, 75*(4), 323–332.

22. Taddei, J. A., Westphal, M. F., Venancio, S., Bogus, C., & Souza, S. (2000). Breastfeeding training for health professionals and resultant changes in breastfeeding duration. *São Paulo Medical Journal, 118*(6), 185–191.

23. Cattaneo, A., & Buzzetti, R. (2001). Effect of rates of breast feeding of training for the Baby Friendly Hospital Initiative. *British Medical Journal, 323,* 1358–1362.

24. Hillenbrand, K. M., & Larsen, P. G. (2002). Effect of an educational intervention about breastfeeding on the knowledge, confidence, and behaviors of pediatric resident physicians. *Pediatrics, 110*(5), e59.

25. Vittoz, J. P., Labarere, J., Castell, M., Durand, M., & Pons, J.C. (2004). Effect of a training program for maternity ward professionals on duration of breastfeeding. *Birth, 31*(4), 302–307.

26. Cantrill, R. M., Creedy, D. K., & Cooke, M. (2003). How midwives learn about breastfeeding. *Australian Journal of Midwifery, 16*(2), 11–16.

27. Sloper, K., McKean, L., & Baum, J. D. (1975). Factors influencing breast feeding. *Archives of Disease in Childhood, 50,* 165–170.

28. Ekström, A., Widstrom, A. M., & Nissen, E. (2005). Process-oriented training in breastfeeding alters attitudes to breastfeeding in health professionals. *Scandinavian Journal of Public Health, 33*(6), 424–431.

29. Iker, C. E., & Mogan, J. (1992). Supplementation of breastfed infants: Does continuing education for nurses make a difference? *Journal of Human Lactation, 8*(3), 131–135.

30. Martens, P. J. (2000). Does breastfeeding education affect nursing staff beliefs, exclusive breastfeeding rates, and Baby-Friendly Hospital Initiative compliance? The experience of a small, rural Canadian hospital. *Journal of Human Lactation, 16*(4), 309–318.

31. World Health Organization and Wellstart International. (1993). *Promoting breast-feeding in health facilities: A short course for administrators and policy makers.* Geneva, Switzerland: World Health Organization, WHO/NHD/96.3).

32. Rea, M. F., Venancio, S. I., Martines, J. C., & Savage, F. (1999). Counselling on breastfeeding: Assessing knowledge and skills. *Bulletin of the World Health Organization, 77*(6), 492–498.

33. Prasad, B., & Costello, A. M. (1995). Impact and sustainability of a "baby friendly" health education intervention at a district hospital in Bihar, India. *British Medical Journal, 310,* 632–623.

CHAPTER

3

Prenatal and Perinatal Education Regarding Infant Feeding

Although this chapter addresses strategies to assure continuity of care in the prenatal care setting, it is our hope that in the future, when breastfeeding is the cultural norm, prenatal breastfeeding education will be less important.

■ Prenatal Breastfeeding Education: Where Should It Occur?

In cultures where breastfeeding is the normal method of infant feeding, education about this essential method begins at birth. Small children see babies fed at the breast and hear their female relatives solving feeding problems. In modern-day North America, the vast majority of women of childbearing age did not grow up witnessing breastfeeding as a common event. Many pregnant women report never having seen a woman breastfeed, and some are not aware of how they were fed themselves as infants. Given the dearth of public knowledge, experience, and ownership of breastfeeding, education about its benefits and management must be retrofitted into our culture. In the United States, expectant families receive infant feeding education (and miseducation) in the context of health care, as well as from their friends and relations.

There have been some initiatives to provide breastfeeding education to the larger community, extending beyond pregnant women to the general population. In New York, breastfeeding education activity packets were designed for inclusion in public school curriculum from kindergarten through grade 12.[1] In 1996, the United States Department of Agriculture's Special Supplemental Nutrition Program for Women, Infants and Children (WIC), which serves low- and moderate-income pregnant and postpartum women, infants and children, inaugurated the Loving Support Makes Breastfeeeding Work campaign to improve breastfeeding rates in the WIC population, which has lower rates of breastfeeding initiation, duration, and exclusivity than occur among families of higher income.[b] One component of Loving Support has been media campaigns to reach

out beyond the mothers and educate the larger community about the importance of breastfeeding and elicit the support of family, friends, coworkers, business leaders, and others in helping families achieve their breastfeeding goals.

The Office on Women's Health of the U.S. Department of Health and Human Services convened a breastfeeding awareness campaign, Babies Were Born to Be Breastfed, in 2004.[2] This campaign, designed to educate the general public about the risks of not breastfeeding, included television and radio public service announcements, print ads, songs, and billboard media. The campaign has been a source of controversy since its inception. In 2007, the *Washington Post* reported that infant formula manufacturers heavily lobbied officials at the Department of Health and Human Services to water down the messages regarding the risks of formula feeding, replacing ads targeted to send messages about linkage between formula use and increased risk of diabetes and childhood cancer with ads linking formula use with increased risk of ear and respiratory tract infections (typically not life-threatening problems).[3]

Aside from individuals who have interacted with the aforementioned programs and campaigns, the bulk of infant feeding education that the average U.S. pregnant woman receives will come through her interactions with the healthcare system, as well as through interactions with her family members and friends. Because the general public is poorly educated about and largely inexperienced with breastfeeding, the information a pregnant woman receives from her family and friends generally includes a web of truth, myths, and rumor. Sadly, the

---

[b] For more information, see: http://www.nal.usda.gov/wicworks/Learning_Center/loving_support.html.

breastfeeding education received by most health professionals is limited at best and often absent from preservice training. Thus, at the current time, breastfeeding education is best achieved by striving to assure the quality and improve the quantity of education disseminated through continuity of care in the healthcare system.

Expectations for Breastfeeding Education in the Health System

Content of Prenatal Education

From the viewpoint of the hospital providing maternity care services, offering appropriate education means that the facility strives to include positive, consistent, evidence-based messages about breastfeeding throughout all prenatal education interactions with expecting families. Topics of education should include the basic benefits of breastfeeding, the importance of exclusive breastfeeding,[c] and the basics of breastfeeding management. See Box 3-1 for self-assessment questions about prenatal education. In addition, women should learn about the breastfeeding-supportive policies and practices in place in the birthing unit, such as immediate skin-to-skin contact after birth, rooming-in, and the avoidance of routine administration of

[c] *Exclusive breastfeeding* refers to the optimal feeding practice of giving the infant no food or drink other than human milk. Note that exclusive breastfeeding is appropriate only to the age of 6 months, after which point breastfeeding should continue and the infant should also receive appropriate complementary foods.

supplements, bottles, and pacifiers (unless medically indicated).

Additionally, pregnant women should receive information about the importance of emotional support during labor, light eating and drinking in labor, nondrug methods of labor pain relief, and the possible effects of analgesia/anesthesia on infant behavior. These issues are related to the amount of energy and ability the woman can bring to the process of interacting and learning to feed her baby in the immediate postpartum period. These topics were added to the international Baby-Friendly Hospital Initiative expectations in the revised documents, and are referred to as the "Mother-Friendly steps."

This issue of the effect of labor and delivery practices on feeding outcomes is an excellent example of the challenge of continuity of care in the hospital The anesthesia and obstetric professionals who provide care during labor are unlikely to observe the feeding difficulties that may ensue from the use of these medications. Similarly, postpartum caregivers may be unaware that labor events and medications may influence postpartum behavior—thus they may not be aware of many factors contributing to feeding difficulties. If the facility does not have a quality improvement process that integrates the horizontal experience of the mother and baby throughout the maternity stay, then the linkage of care practices with feeding outcomes may be invisible to the system. It is also important to educate maternity staff regarding the potential effects of medications on infant feeding.

Delivering Prenatal Education

Ideally, women will receive educational messages throughout their prenatal and perinatal

---

Box 3-1   **Self-Assessment Questions**

The following questions have been modified from the WHO/BFHI self-assessment tool. To see the original, go to http://who.int/nutrition/topics/BFHI_Revised_Section_4.pdf.

Are pregnant women informed about the importance and management of breastfeeding?

    If so, describe how this is accomplished and what the teaching points are.

Do prenatal records indicate whether breastfeeding has been discussed with pregnant women?

    If so, what is written in the records? How much detail is given?

Does prenatal education, including both that provided orally and in written form, cover key topics related to the importance and management of breastfeeding?

    If so, what are the key topics? What written materials are used?

Are pregnant women protected from oral or written promotion of and group instruction on artificial feeding?

    What policies offer this protection? How are they audited?

Are pregnant women able to describe the risks of giving supplements while breastfeeding in the first 6 months?

What are the risks that are routinely conveyed to mothers?

Are pregnant women able to describe the importance of early and uninterrupted skin-to-skin contact between mothers and babies?

Are pregnant women able to describe the importance of rooming-in with their babies?

---

experiences with the health system. If the birth facility employs the obstetric care providers who have privileges on the maternity unit, then the facility should require breast-feeding counseling and education during specific prenatal care interactions as well as during childbirth education. If the facility does not employ the prenatal care providers, it should recommend the coverage of breast-feeding topics in prenatal care to all providers with obstetric privileges. The facility should integrate breastfeeding messages into all pre-natal education curricula, from early preg-nancy classes through childbirth education. Short, positive messages, similar to the sound bites popular in political campaigns, help to build a sense of normalcy around breastfeed-ing. Any educational materials disseminated to women must be free of messages that pro-mote artificial feeding.

Every care provider who interacts with the pregnant/childbearing woman should of-fer targeted messages about breastfeeding. Obstetric care providers can integrate breast-feeding messages by simple interactions, such as mentioning the darkening of the areolae during pregnancy as a sign of the body's prep-aration for breastfeeding. Childbirth educa-tors can mention the increase in breast size as a sign that the body is preparing for breast-feeding, or discuss the importance of skin-to-skin contact during the first hour after birth in beginning breastfeeding. Mentioning breastfeeding in this way helps to reinforce the reality that breastfeeding is the natural consequence of pregnancy—women may have a cognitive choice in terms of how they feed their babies, but to their endocrine and physiologic systems, lactation is a mandate, not an option.

The U.S. Breastfeeding Committee has noted that breastfeeding should be portrayed as "normal, desirable, and achievable."[4] The language sometimes used to describe breast-feeding often uses terms such as *the gold stan-dard* and *optimal*. Many childbearing women may be put off by those terms, which signify something above and beyond their means, or costly to provide. When healthcare provid-ers discuss breastfeeding in a matter-of-fact way, women may think differently about it, perhaps thinking, "My doctor or nurse thinks I could breastfeed—maybe I'll try!"

■ Evidence for the Effect of Prenatal Breastfeeding Education

In 2003, the U.S. Preventive Services Task Force (USPSTF) released recommendations on the promotion of breastfeeding, includ-ing an evidence review of primary care in-terventions to promote breastfeeding,[5] and found that some commonly implemented interventions were not supported by suf-ficient evidence of efficacy although other interventions had fair or good evidence of efficacy.

The USPSTF concluded that there is insufficient evidence to recommend for or against the following interventions:

- brief education and counseling by primary care providers during routine visits
- peer counseling used alone and initiated from the clinical setting in industrialized countries

Also, the evidence for the effectiveness of written materials suggests no significant ben-efit when written materials are used alone, and there is mixed evidence of incremental benefit when written materials are used in combination with other interventions.

However, the USPSTF found fair evi-dence that programs in primary care settings that combined breastfeeding education with behaviorally oriented counseling were associated with increased rates of breastfeeding initiation and its continuation for up to 3 months, although effects beyond 3 months were uncertain. Effective programs generally involved the following:

- at least one extended individual or group session
- following structured protocols
- practical, behavioral skills training and problem solving in addition to didactic instruction

The sessions were led by specially trained nurses or lactation specialists and usually lasted 30 to 90 minutes. As a result, the USPSTF recommends that clinicians routinely provide this kind of structured breastfeeding education and behavioral counseling programs to promote breastfeeding.

The USPSTF found that providing ongoing breastfeeding support, through in-person visits or telephone contacts with providers or counselors, increased the proportion of women continuing to breastfeed for up to 6 months. Peer counselor and mother-to-mother support programs initiated in community-based WIC programs are an effective strategy for promoting and supporting breastfeeding, especially in combination with lactation specialists and when the peer counselors are given sufficient time (at least 45 minutes) to provide education and support.[6]

The USPSTF did not evaluate visiting nurse or public health nursing programs designed to promote or support breastfeeding. In addition, the USPSTF did not consider the impact of improved maternity care practices on breastfeeding outcomes. The impact of a nurse appraising a breastfeeding, either in the hospital or in the mother's home, has been found to be an effective strategy to increase breastfeeding duration,[7] and mothers expect nurses to fill this role.[8] One research team noted that "Prenatal breastfeeding education strategies may affect women's breastfeeding intentions, but strategies focusing on the early postpartum period can assist women in executing those intentions."[9]

The impact of implementing improved maternity care practices such as those embedded in the WHO/UNICEF Baby-Friendly Hospital Initiative's *Ten Steps to Successful Breastfeeding*[d] have been studied in a randomized, controlled trial and found to improve breastfeeding initiation as well as duration at 6 months and 1 year.[10] In addition, mothers' experiences of maternity practices have been examined with the finding that the more steps of *The Ten Steps to Successful Breastfeeding* the mother reported experiencing, the longer her breastfeeding duration.[11]

In order to optimize breastfeeding in the United States, private and public sectors must work together to promote, protect, and support this valuable foundation of good health. Nurses should work to ensure that policies, programs, protocols, and practices are based on evidence-based research such as those suggested by the USPSTF. Hospital and community committees as well as professional nursing organizations are an excellent venue for nurses to work to develop evidence-based policies and programs. Professional organizations of nurses endorse evidence-based

---

[d] Administered in the United States by Baby-Friendly USA, 327 Quaker Meeting House Road, East Sandwich, MA 02537. Web site: info@babyfriendlyusa.org.

practices that oblige work sites to adopt them. Nurses should participate in interdisciplinary healthcare system committees in order to advance continuity of care through evidence-based policies and practice.

In the report of evidence reviewed to guide the USPSTF recommendation discussed previously, Guise, Palda, Westhoff, Chan, Helfand, and Lieu found "encouraging evidence that educational programs and support services … can improve breastfeeding initiation and duration rates in the United States and other developed countries."[12] Of all the education methods examined, the review found the best outcomes for prenatal education sessions "that review the benefits of breastfeeding, principles of lactation, myths, common problems, solutions and skills training appear to have the greatest single effect. One woman would successfully initiate and maintain breastfeeding for up to 3 months for every 3 to 5 women that attended educational sessions."[13]

In order for educational messages to be received by women, it is crucial that they are offered excellent communication and counseling skills. Taveras, Li, Grummer-Strawn, Richardson, Marshall, Rego, and colleagues identified prenatal care providers who stated that they usually or always discussed breastfeeding duration during prenatal care.[14] The researchers then interviewed women after a prenatal visit, and found that only 16% of mothers reported that their prenatal care provider had discussed breastfeeding duration with them. This finding suggests that it is important that rote educational messages be avoided; rather discussion should be client centered and specific to the individual woman.

Reliance on written material is not recommended, as research indicates no positive effect of written material alone on choosing breastfeeding.[15] If written information is given, it should be free of references to breast milk substitutes and should not contain information about the use of substitutes. Howard, Howard, Lawrence, Andresen, DeBlieck, and Weitzman have identified that prenatal education packets provided by a formula company negatively impact the breastfeeding in the first 2 weeks.[16] The authors of this study concluded, "Educational materials about infant feeding should support unequivocally breast-feeding as optimal nutrition for infants; formula promotion products should be eliminated from prenatal settings."[17]

Evidence for the "Mother-Friendly" Steps

As mentioned above, in its 2006 revision of the Baby-Friendly Hospital Initiative, the World Health Organization and UNICEF urged the inclusion in prenatal education of messages regarding the importance of emotional support during labor, light eating and drinking in labor, non-drug methods of labor pain relief, and the possible effects of analgesia/anesthesia on infant behavior. This section will review what is know of the effect of these experiences on maternal-infant bonding and breastfeeding.

Research regarding the effects of *emotional support during labor* has blossomed in recent decades. A Cochrane review[18] found that women who received continuous support during labor were more likely to give birth vaginally (rather than via cesarean) and to do so without forceps or vacuum assist. Additionally, supported women were less likely to use medications for pain relief, had slightly shorter labors, and were more likely to be satisfied with their care. The authors noted that labor support appeared to be more effective when was provided by someone who was it not a member of the hospital staff.

Medications used for pain relief during labor can alter the behavior of the infant and may decrease the mother's ability to respond to her baby in the immediate postpartum. Writing on behalf of the Academy of Breastfeeeding Medicine's Protocol Committee, Montgomery and Hale[19] state:

"Use of pharmacologic agents for pain relief in labor and postpartum may improve outcomes by relieving suffering during labor and allowing mothers to recover from birth, especially Cesarean birth, with minimal interference from pain. However, these methods also may affect the course of labor and the neurobehavioral state of the neonate, and have adverse effects on breastfeeding initiation."

Montgomery and Hale go on to review the potential impact of several categories of medications on feeding abilities, and recommend that women receive informed consent in the prenatal period prior to the onset of labor.

Evidence regarding the use of non-drug pain relief methods was reviewed in 2007 by Leslie, Romano, and Woolley on behalf of the Coalition for Improving Maternity Services,[20] finding good quality evidence for:

- the use of touch or massage in decreasing pain and anxiety, among other effects;
- for the role of hypnosis in greater maternal satisfaction with treatment and reduced need for augmentation with oxytocin, among other effects; and

- for lack of negative outcomes associated with use of hydrotherapy during labor.

Leslie, Romano, and Wooley also found good quality evidence linkage between:

- use of opiod drugs in labor and respiratory distress in the newborn, less alertness in the newborn in the first hours after birth, and increased risk of delayed onset of successful breastfeeding.[21]

■ Common Barriers to Delivering Prenatal Breastfeeding Education and Strategies to Overcome Them

In the U.S. healthcare system, *fragmentation of care* complicates the delivery of perinatal education. In health systems where the prenatal care providers are not employed by the facilities where they deliver, the facility may have little control over the content of prenatal education delivered by the provider, and it may have little interaction with pregnant women until birth is imminent. Health maintenance organizations and public health system hospitals have an advantage in the ability to provide seamless education throughout the pregnancy, with some education opportunities even prior to conception in some systems. Hospital systems have overcome this barrier through a variety of methods, including:

- Creating a working group with representatives of providers in the community to develop or adapt the following:
  - a prenatal booklet about breastfeeding and breastfeeding promotion in-

terventions that can be distributed through all affiliated prenatal care practitioners

- ◆ a teaching checklist for obstetric care providers that provides talking points about breastfeeding for each prenatal visit

- ◆ waiting room educational resources (e.g., posters and videos) to pique women's interest

- Encouraging the use of pregnancy-centering groups to build a community of women with similar due dates.[22] Many positive outcomes of centering groups have been cited, including knowledge of pregnancy health,[23] as well as satisfaction with prenatal care.[24] Creation of these groups offers a natural place for breastfeeding education in a cost- and time-effective manner.

- Inviting community breastfeeding resources such as La Leche League, Nursing Mothers Council, WIC breastfeeding specialists and peer counselors, and freelance lactation care providers to contribute education to pregnant women.

A second challenge to implementing prenatal breastfeeding education is *poor attendance at prenatal classes.* Many birth facilities report that 20% or fewer of their delivering families attend any educational offerings. To overcome this barrier, birthing facilities have employed strategies such as:

- Presenting concise breastfeeding messages visually through posters and videos placed at ultrasonography, laboratories, and other locations where pregnant women may be waiting, as well as in obstetric care waiting rooms.

- Including infant feeding education in regular childbirth classes, rather than providing an optional class at the end of the series.

- Offering childbirth/breastfeeding education in weekend, lunchtime, and electronic formats to allow working parents flexibility.

- Inviting other community breastfeeding resource people to provide education on-site during waiting time.

Yet another challenge to prenatal education may be the *variable knowledge base and comfort of prenatal care providers* and other key staff with breastfeeding and breastfeeding education. It is important that the information women receive from different care providers is consistent. It is also crucial that educators appear comfortable with breastfeeding—otherwise staff may inadvertently send mixed messages to pregnant women. Implementation of staff and provider education, as discussed in Chapter 2, is thus an important precursor to improving prenatal education. In order to assure provider comfort with breastfeeding, training sessions should include adequate opportunities to role play education and counseling techniques and practice correct responses to frequently asked breastfeeding questions.

Resources

American College of Obstetricians and Gynecologists. (2007). Breastfeeding: Maternal and infant aspects [Special report from ACOG]. *ACOG Clinical Review, 12*(1, Suppl), 1S–16S.

Declercq, E. R., Sakala, C., Corry, M. P., Applebaum, S., Risher, P. (2002, October). *Listening to Mothers: Report of the first national survey of women's childbearing experiences.* New York: Maternity Center Association.

Lamaze Institute for Normal Birth. (2007). *Six Care Practices that Support Normal Birth*. Retrieved at http://www.lamaze.org/AboutLamaze/LamazeInstituteforNormalBirth/tabid/171/Default.aspx on 12/1/07.

Leslie, M. S., Romano, A., & Woolley, D. (2007, Winter Supplement). Step 7: Educates staff in nondrug methods of pain relief and does not promote use of analgesic, anesthetic drugs. *The Journal of Perinatal Education*, 16(1): 65S–73S.

Leslie, M. S., & Storton, S. (2007, Winter Supplement) Step 1: Offers all birthing mothers unrestricted access to birth companions, labor support, professional midwifery care. *The Journal of Perinatal Education*, 16(1), 10S–19S.

Montgomery, A., Hale, T. W., & Academy of Breastfeeding Medicine Protocol Committee. (2006, Winter). ABM clinical protocol #15: Analgesia and anesthesia for the breastfeeding mother. *Breastfeeding Medicine*, 1(4), 271–277.

Smith, L. J. (2007). Impact of birthing practices on the breastfeeding dyad. *Journal of Midwifery & Women's Health*, 52(6), 621–630.

References

1. New York State Department of Health, Bureau of Women's Health. (2004). *A breastfeeding education activity packet for grades K–12: A practical classroom tool*. Albany, NY: Author. Retrieved September 14, 2007, from http://www.health.state.ny.us/community/pregnancy/breastfeeding/main.htm.

2. The National Women's Health Information Center. (2007). *National breastfeeding awareness campaign: Babies were born to be breastfed*. Retrieved on September 18, 2007, from http://www.4women.gov/breastfeeding/index.cfm?page=Campaign

3. Kaufman, M., & Lee, C. (2007, August 31). HHS toned down breastfeeding ads: Formula industry urged softer campaign. *The Washington Post*, A01.

4. United States Breastfeeding Committee. (2001). *Breastfeeding in the United States: A national agenda*. Rockville, MD: U.S. Department of Health and Human Services, Health Resources and Services Administration, Maternal Child Health Bureau, 11.

5. Guise, J. M., Palda, V., Westhoff, C., Chan, B. K., Helfand, M., Lieu, T. A., et al. (2003). The effectiveness of primary care-based interventions to promote breastfeeding: Systematic evidence review and meta-analysis for the U.S. Preventive

Services Task Force. *Annals of Family Medicine, 1*(2), 70–78.

6. Grummer-Strawn, L. M., Rice, S. P., Dugas, K., Clark, L. D., & Benton-Davis, S. (1997, March). An evaluation of breastfeeding promotion through counseling in Mississippi WIC clinics. *Maternal Child Health Journal, 1*(1), 35–42.

7. Kuan, L. W., Britto, M., Decolongon, J., Schoetker, P. J., Atherton, H. D., & Kotagal, U. R. (1999, September). Health system factors contributing to breastfeeding success. *Pediatrics, 104*(3), e29.

8. Gill, S. L. (2001). The little things: Perceptions of breastfeeding support. *Journal of Obstetric, Gynecologic, and Neonatal Nursing, 30*(4), 401–409.

9. Ahluwalia, I. B., Tessaro, I., Grummer-Strawn, L. M., MacGowan, C., & Benton-Davis, S. (2000). Georgia's breastfeeding promotion program for low-income women. *Pediatrics, 105*(6), e85.

10. Kramer, M. S., Chalmers, B., Hodnett, E. D., Sevkovskaya, Z., Dzikovich, I., Shapiro, S., et al. (2000). Promotion of breastfeeding intervention trial (PROBIT): A cluster-randomized trial in the Republic of Belarus. Design, follow-up, and data validation. *Advances in Experimental Medicine and Biology, 478*, 327–345.

11. DiGirolamo, A. M., Grummer-Strawn, L. M., & Fein, S. (2001). Maternity care practices: Implications for breastfeeding. *Birth, 28*, 2.

12. Guise, J. M., Palda, V., Westhoff, C., Chan, B. K., Helfand, M., Lieu, T. A., et al. (2003). The effectiveness of primary care-based interventions to promote breastfeeding: Systematic evidence review and meta-analysis for the U.S. Preventive Services Task Force. *Annals of Family Medicine, 1*(2), 76.

13. Guise, J. M., Palda, V., Westhoff, C., Chan, B. K., Helfand, M., Lieu, T. A., et al. (2003). The effectiveness of primary care-based interventions to promote breastfeeding: Systematic evidence review and meta-analysis for the U.S. Preventive Services Task Force. *Annals of Family Medicine, 1*(2), 75.

14. Taveras, E. M., Li, R., Grummer-Strawn, L., Richardson, M., Marshall, R., Rego, V. H., et al. (2004). Mothers' and clinicians' perspectives on breastfeeding counseling during routine preventive visits. *Pediatrics, 113*(5), e405–e411.

15. Guise, J. M., Palda, V., Westhoff, C., Chan, B. K., Helfand, M., Lieu, T. A., et al. (2003). The effectiveness of primary care-based interventions to promote breastfeeding: Systematic evidence review and meta-analysis for the U.S. Preventive

Services Task Force. *Annals of Family Medicine, 1*(2), 70–78.

16. Howard, C. R., Howard, F. M., Lawrence, R. A., Andresen, E., DeBlieck, E., & Weitzman, M. (2002). The effect on breastfeeding of physicians' office-based prenatal formula advertising. *Obstetrics and Gynecology, 95*(2), 296–303.

17. Howard, C. R., Howard, F. M., Lawrence, R. A., Andresen, E., DeBlieck, E., & Weitzman, M. (2002). The effect on breastfeeding of physicians' office-based prenatal formula advertising. *Obstetrics and Gynecology, 95*(2), 296.

18. Hodnett, E. D., Gates, S., Hofmeyr, G. J., & Sakala, C. (2003). Continuous support for women during childbirth. *Cochrane Database of Systematic Reviews*, (3),CD003766. DOI: 10.1002/14651858. CD003766.pub2

19. Montgomery, A., Hale, T. W., & Academy of Breastfeeding Medicine Protocol Committee. (2006, Winter). ABM clinical protocol #15: analgesia and anesthesia for the breastfeeding mother. *Breastfeeding Medicine, 1*(4), 271.

20. Leslie, M. S., Romano, A., Woolley, D. (2007, Winter Supplement) Step 7: Educates staff in non-drug methods of pain relief and does not promote use of analgesic, anesthetic drugs. *The Journal of Perinatal Education,* 16(1): 65S–73S.

21. Leslie, M. S., Romano, A., Woolley, D. (2007, Winter Supplement) Step 7: Educates staff in non-drug methods of pain relief and does not promote use of analgesic, anesthetic drugs. *The Journal of Perinatal Education,* 16(1): 68S–69.

22. Rising, S. S., Kennedy, H. P., & Klima, C. S. (2004). Redesigning prenatal care through centering pregnancy. *Journal of Midwifery and Women's Health, 49*(5), 398–404.

23. Baldwin, K. A. (2006). Comparison of selected outcomes of centering pregnancy. *Journal of Midwifery and Women's Health, 51*(4), 266–272.

24. Grady, M. A., & Bloom, K. C. (2004). Pregnancy outcomes of adolescents enrolled in a centering pregnancy program. *Journal of Midwifery and Women's Health, 49*(5), 412– 420.

Getting Breastfeeding Off to a Good Start

The First Hour After Birth

Ten Steps to Successful Breastfeeding
A Joint WHO/UNICEF Statement[a]

Every facility providing maternity services and care for newborn infants should:

1. Have a written breastfeeding policy that is routinely communicated to all healthcare staff.
2. Train all healthcare staff in skills necessary to implement this policy.
3. Inform all pregnant women about the benefits and management of breastfeeding.
4. **Help mothers initiate breastfeeding within a half-hour of birth. (US, one hour)**
5. Show mothers how to breastfeed, and how to maintain lactation even if they should be separated from their infants.
6. Give newborn infants no food or drink other than breastmilk unless *medically* indicated.
7. Practice rooming in—allow mothers and infants to remain together—24 hours a day.
8. Encourage breastfeeding on demand.
9. Give no artificial teats (US, nipples) or pacifiers (also called dummies or soothers) to breastfeeding infants.
10. Foster the establishment of breastfeeding support groups and refer mothers to them on discharge from the hospital or clinic.

[a] World Health Organization. (1989). *Protecting, promoting and supporting breast-feeding: The special role of maternity services.* Geneva, Switzerland: World Health Organization, p. iv

More maternity care facilities are experiencing the magic of skin-to-skin contact in the first hour. Our colleague, video ethnographer Kajsa Brimdyr, tells us that when she was filming a mother and baby skin-to-skin after a cesarean birth recently, she had to turn her video camera's screen so that the surgical staff closing the mother's abdomen could glance at the baby while they worked. Seeing the baby's innate capabilities, and the beauty of the unspoken language of the mother and baby's first meeting, is a wondrous and important experience not to be missed even by veteran maternity caregivers.[1]

■ The Importance of Mother-Baby Contact during the First Hour after Birth

The first hour after birth is a crucial time for the mother and baby to begin their postpartum relationship. Entrenched delivery routines and procedures are often at odds with biological needs during this period. The common goal of the healthcare workers involved in peripartum care is to assess the baby, assess the mother, and care for and stabilize both. Because our system sees the newborn as a *pediatric* patient and the mother as an *obstetric* patient, the urge is to care for them separately and reunite them when both are deemed stable. Nothing could be further from the biologic imperative. In order for baby and mother to recover from the birth and stabilize, they should do so as a unit. Take the example of immediate suckling. When the newborn first suckles at the breast, he receives tiny amounts of colostrum, which provides small amounts of nutrition, paints the gut wall with the appropriate immunoglobulins to protect him against specific pathogens in the mother/baby environment, and prompts passage of meconium. The experience of nuzzling, licking, and suckling produces an outpouring of hormones that stabilize baby's blood sugar, reduce the stress response, and relax the baby. When the baby nuzzles, licks, and suckles, the mother's body responds by releasing hormones that contract the uterus, slowing blood loss, and reducing the mother's stress response, further relaxing her, as well as driving her to attend to, stroke, and bond with her baby.

We know about the dangers of separating newborn animals from their mothers. But we do not seem to recognize that there is negative effect to separating human newborns from their mothers in the sensitive period after birth, unless there is extreme medical instability. For example, the preterm baby, the baby with respiratory or cardiac problems, or the mother who experiences hemorrhage should, of course, be attended to as appropriate. However, the vast majority of mothers and babies can be cared for together in the first hours after birth.

Ideally, immediately after birth, the baby is gently dried, visually examined, and laid on his mother's abdomen. The baby is dried to slow evaporative heat loss as he learns to maintain his body temperature outside his mother's body. The warmth of her skin and the sound of her heartbeat and familiar voice appear to comfort the baby as he experiences a new, brighter, noisier, less fluid-filled environment. There is no reason to suspect that baby will become cold on his mother's body; as long as the baby is dried, the mother's body will warm him. If the mother is cold, she and the baby should be covered, leaving the baby's head free of the blanket.

Fascinating research from Sweden has identified that, when allowed to lie skin to skin with their mothers for the first hour or 2 after birth, newborn babies can find the breast and initiate suckling without any help from their mothers.[2,3] Phyllis and Marshall Klaus have encapsulated the importance of the first hour:

> There is something special about the first hour of life. Parents have waited many months to see their baby and

surprisingly when the baby is born, he or she is in a special state of alertness—called State Four, the quiet state of consciousness, ready to meet its parents, and is especially interested in the mother's and father's face.

In this special state, the baby's eyes are wide open, the baby is quiet. The baby has heard and remembers the mother's voice from uterine life and will distinguish her voice from other women's voices, and 80% of babies remember the father's voice. The baby is warmed by the mother's chest and soothed by the mother's touch. This quiet time together helps the transition from uterine life to the outside world.

This special state in the infant lasts for 30 to 45 minutes or longer. All sorts of exchanges between the mother and infant are going on. The baby is taking-in the mother through many senses as is the mother learning about her baby. The baby is becoming familiar with the mother's smell and within a few days will pick out his or her mother's breast pad from other women's breast pads. This is related to the particular smell of one's own mother not her milk.

As the baby gazes in the mother's face he is recording a memory of her face so that if he is tested with a picture of his mother's face and other women's faces four hours later, he will choose his mother's face over and over again.

The mother is taking in her baby also, by touch, smell, as well as sight.

Curiously, if she is tested a few hours later to pick out her baby from two others, she will know her baby by touch and smell within one day.[4]

■ Expectations for Care in the First Hour after Birth

All healthy, full-term babies should be placed skin to skin (STS) with their mother, wearing nothing but perhaps a diaper and a hat, immediately after birth, and held there continuously until the end of the first feeding, and longer if possible. Staff should offer assistance during this period to help the parents learn and respond to the infant's feeding cues.

In the event of cesarean birth, the baby should be placed skin to skin with its mother as soon as she is able to safely respond to and hold her baby. How long this takes may be a function of the amount and type of anesthesia she received. Staff should offer assistance with learning and responding to feeding cues during this time. It is also possible for staff members to safeguard the baby at the breast before the mother is fully recovered.

While the baby is skin to skin with the mother, staff should be observing mother and baby, just as they would if the two were apart.

STS contact during the first hour of life is recommended, regardless of the feeding intention of the mother.

In its 2006 revision of the Baby-Friendly Hospital Initiative, the World Health Organization and UNICEF added clarification regarding the interpretation of Step 4 of the Ten Steps to Successful Breastfeeding. The following language appears in the Hospital Self-Appraisal Tool:

"STEP 4. Help mothers initiate breastfeeding within a half-hour of birth. This Step is now interpreted as: Place babies in STS contact with their mothers immediately following birth for at least an hour and encourage mothers to recognize when their babies are ready to breastfeed, offering help if needed."[5]

■ Evidence for Skin to Skin Care in the Immediate Postpartum Period

Fascinating research from around the globe identifies several beneficial aspects of skin contact in the postpartum period.

Increased Infant Survival

Research from Ghana indicates that early initiation of breastfeeding is associated with improved infant survival in this developing country. The study population included more than 10,000 newborn infants and indicated that 22% of neonatal deaths could be averted if breastfeeding were initiated in the first hour of life.[6] The application of this finding to the Western world is unknown; however, it does underscore the importance of early mother–baby contact and early breastfeeding as a public health issue, rather than a nice thing that mothers and babies can do.

Decreased Stress and Increased Homeostasis for the Baby

Researchers have identified that early skin contact in the first hours of life improves the baby's motor skill coordination. The first hours after birth are a time of intense transition for the baby. Maintaining homeostasis (body balance) is a challenge for the newborn, who must learn to breathe, regulate body temperature, heart, and respiratory rates, and process many new sensations from the extrauterine world. Ferber and Makhoul demonstrated that infants held STS during the first hour of life had more flexed and fewer extended movements (indicating less stress) and maintained restful sleep longer in the first 6 hours of life.[7] The authors conclude that extended STS contact "shortly after delivery might be used as a beneficial clinical intervention to reduce the stress associated with birth and to pave the pathway for the increasingly independent self-regulation of the newborn in face of the inevitable extra-uterine bombardment with environmental stimulus."[8] STS care should be practiced with all mother/baby couplets, not just those planning to breastfeed, as all mothers and babies will benefit from the stress reduction and bonding promoted by extended skin contact.

Improved Temperature Regulation

Several research studies have indicated that STS care is as effective as or more effective at helping babies maintain body temperature than incubator care. In England, a trial of more than 200 mother/baby couplets found that the baby's mean body temperature 1 hour after birth was higher with STS contact than with routine care.[9]

Improved Breastfeeding Outcomes and Maternal Attachment Behavior

A Cochrane review of early STS contact identified statistically significant effects of early

STS on breastfeeding continuation at 1 and 4 months of life (odds ratio 1.82) as well as trends toward increased scores of maternal affectionate love/touch during observed feedings, and maternal attachment behavior with early STS.[10] Babies held STS cried for a shorter length of time, and late preterm infants cared for in this way had better cardiorespiratory stability in one trial of STS care. The review found no adverse effects of STS care.

Spontaneous Breastfeeding

During STS care, babies often initiate feeding on their own. Widström, Ransjo-Arvidsön, Christensson, Matthiesen, Winberg, and Uvnäs-Moberg were the first to report that infants demonstrate a predictable pattern of behavior when held STS on their mothers' chests in the first hour after birth.[11] These behaviors culminate in the baby locating, attaching to, and suckling from the mother's nipple. Babies began moving toward the breast after the first several minutes of life, with suckling beginning around the end of the first hour. Righard and Alade found that these behaviors were most likely to be seen when the infant had not been separated from the mother for cleaning and measurement, and that babies born after unmedicated labor were more likely to find the nipple and suckle than those whose mothers had received pain medication during labor.[12] The latter research study reported that babies who were not separated from their mothers during the first hour were more likely to suckle correctly during subsequent feedings. The first feeding appears to have a powerful patterning effect for subsequent feeds.

■ Common Barriers to Optimal Practice in the First Hour of Life and Strategies to Overcome Barriers

A prominent barrier is the *routine practice of mother–baby separation* in the first hour for examination and cleaning of the baby and stabilization of the mother and baby. Maternity staff have many tasks to complete in the first hour of life, and many perceive it is best to just run through the checklist, do all the procedures, and *then* leave mother and baby together. This is done without awareness of the importance of those first minutes and hours for the development of the maternal–infant bond and the stabilization of the baby.

A helpful strategy to overcome this barrier is to review the guidance of the American College of Obstetricians and Gynecologists (ACOG), the American Academy of Pediatrics (AAP), and the Academy of Breastfeeding Medicine (ABM) regarding the appropriate management of mother and baby in the first hour.

In 2007, the ACOG published a clinical review of breastfeeding.[13] This document states:

> The immediate postpartum period should allow the woman and her newborn to experience optimal bonding with immediate physical contact, preferably skin to skin. Separation may lead to complications such as hypothermia and hypoglycemia, increasing the likelihood of supplementation. The initial feeding should occur as soon as possible, preferably

in the first hour when the baby is awake, alert, and ready to suckle. The longer the interval between birth and the first feeding, the more likely the use of supplementation. Newborn eye prophylaxis, weighing, measuring and other such examinations should be deferred until after the first feeding or until they can take place without separating the infant from the mother. Such procedures usually can be performed later in the mother's room.[14]

The 2005 AAP policy statement on breastfeeding advises:

Healthy infants should be placed and remain in direct skin-to-skin contact with their mothers immediately after delivery until the first feeding is accomplished.

- The alert, healthy newborn infant is capable of latching on to a breast without specific assistance within the first hour after birth. Dry the infant, assign Apgar scores, and perform the initial physical assessment while the infant is with the mother. The mother is an optimal heat source for the infant. Delay weighing, measuring, bathing, needle-sticks, and eye prophylaxis until after the first feeding is completed. Infants affected by maternal medications may require assistance for effective latch-on. Except under unusual circumstances, the newborn infant should remain with the mother during the recovery period.[15]

ABM's protocol for peripartum breastfeeding management states:

The healthy newborn can be given directly to the mother for skin-to-skin contact until the first feeding is accomplished. The infant may be dried and assigned Apgar scores and the initial physical assessment performed as the infant is placed with the mother. Such contact provides the infant optimal physiologic stability, warmth, and opportunities for the first feeding. Delaying procedures such as weighing, measuring, and administering vitamin K and eye prophylaxis (up to an hour) enhances early parent–infant interaction. Infants are to be put to the breast as soon after birth as feasible for both mother and infant (within an hour of birth). This is to be initiated in either the delivery room or recovery room, and every mother is to be instructed in proper breastfeeding technique.[16]

The Association of Women's Health, Obstetric and Neonatal Nurses (AWHONN) indicates that, among other responsibilities for the nurse at the time of birth, nurses should "Promote non-separation of mother-baby in postpartum period . . . [and] Assure breastfeeding initiation in the immediate postpartum period, barring maternal or neonatal complications."[17]

Another common barrier is the staff perception that *routine procedures* (e.g., bathing, warming, observation) have priority over breastfeeding in the first hour of life or that these procedures should be done first in order to allow the mother and baby time to relax together. The pressure to complete the many tasks that must be completed in the admission of the infant may take precedence if staff do not understand how crucial the first hour is to the establishment of a solid mother–baby bond. The AAP, ABM, and ACOG statements cited previously clearly indicate that routine procedures should be delayed in favor of immediate mother–baby contact.

Education can help overcome this barrier. Seeing the newborn's innate abilities to find the breast can be revolutionary to many professionals. Typically, newborns are swaddled tightly in the first hour, and are less able to demonstrate their abilities to move about on the mother's abdomen, seeking, finding, and latching to her nipples. Veteran care providers who have witnessed this ability have been heard to say, "I had no idea that babies knew where to go, and what to do." Two excellent video presentations of this interaction can be found on the resource list for this chapter.

A common barrier may be the assumption that skin to skin is reserved for the healthy full-term baby, and may not be available for the immature, sick, or uncoordinated baby who is struggling with state or motor regulation. Actually, STS contact has been demonstrated to assist premature and ill babies in regulating body functions and motor skills. A special kind of STS contact, known as Kangaroo Mother Care (KMC), is practiced in many special care units around the world. The KMC technique keeps the baby vertically upright between the mother's breasts and closely to her body. Research indicates that early and continuous KMC increases breastfeeding success.[18] Therefore STC contact and KMC should be encouraged as early and continuously as possible in the care of the preterm and ill infant as well as among healthy term infants.

Conducting small-scale research can be a powerful way to document and change the effects of delivery room routines. Take, for example, the situation where unit management wants to implement immediate skin-to-skin contact after birth, but there is concern among some staff members that babies will become hypothermic. One way to address this concern would be to create a small-scale observational study in which staff would collect the data on body temperature management of the next 10 babies held skin to skin and the following 10 babies cared for in the routine manner. Looking at the results of this study may help to allay fears and identify potential problems with new care methods. This method allows everyone involved the opportunity to be more analytical and less reactionary about the proposed change.

Resources

Academy of Breastfeeeding Medicine. (n.d.). Protocol #5: Peripartum breastfeeding management for the healthy mother and infant at term. Available at http://bfmed.org/ace-files/protocol/peripartum.pdf.

American Academy of Pediatrics, Section on Breastfeeding. (2005). Breastfeeding and the use of human milk. *Pediatrics, 115:*496–506.

American College of Nurse-Midwives. (2005). Position statement: Breastfeeding. Silver Spring, MD: ACNM. Available at http://www.midwife.org/site-Files/position/Breastfeeding_05.pdf.

American College of Obstetricians and Gynecologists. (2007). Breastfeeding: Maternal and infant aspects. Special report from ACOG. *ACOG Clinical Review, 12*(1, Suppl), 1S–16S.

Anderson, G. C., Moore, E., Hepworth, J., & Bergman, N. (2003). Early skin-to-skin contact for mothers and their healthy newborn infants. *Cochrane Database of Systematic Reviews,* (2):CD003519.

Association of Women's Health, Obstetric and Neonatal Nurses. (1999). *Breastfeeding: Clinical position statement.* Washington, DC: AWHONN.

Association of Women's Health, Obstetric and Neonatal Nurses. (1999). *Role of the nurse in the promotion of breastfeeding.* Washington, DC: AWHONN.

Gangal, P. (Ed.). (2007). *Breast crawl: Initiation of breastfeeding by breast crawl.* Mumbai, India: UNICEF Maharashtra. Retrieved on September 17, 2007, from http://breastcrawl.org/pdf/breastcrawl.pdf.

Ransjö-Arvidson, A. B., Matthiesen, A. S., Lilja, G., Nissen, E., Widström, A. M., & Uvnäs-Moberg, K. (2001). Maternal analgesia during labor disturbs newborn behavior: Effects on breastfeeding, temperature, and crying. *Birth, 28*(1), 5–12.

Righard, L., & Alade, M. O. (1990). Effect of delivery room routines on success of first breast-feed. *Lancet, 336*(8723), 1105–1107.

Video Presentations on Infant Self-Attachment Behavior

Righard, L. (n.d.) *Delivery Self-Attachment.* Available from Health Education Associates, www.healthed.cc and Geddes Productions: http://www.geddesproduction.com/breast-feeding-delivery-selfattachment.html

Widström, A.-M., Ransjö-Arvidson, A. B., & Christensson, K. (2007). *Breastfeeding is … Baby's Choice* [Videotape]. Stockholm, Sweden: BKG Productions. Available in the United States and Canada from Health Education Associates, www.healthed.cc.

References

1. Brimdyr, K. Personal communication, 12/15/07.
2. Widström, A. M., Wahlberg, V., & Matthiesen, A. S. (1990). Short-term effects of early suckling and touch of the nipple on maternal behaviour. *Early Human Development, 21*(3), 153–163.
3. Righard, L., & Alade, M. O. (1990). Effect of delivery room routines on success of first breastfeed. *Lancet, 336*(8723), 1105–1107.
4. Klaus, P., & Klaus, M. (2007). Preface. In P. Gangal (Ed.), *Breast crawl: Initiation of breastfeeding by breast crawl* (pp. 7–8). Mumbai, India: UNICEF Maharashtra. Retrieved on September 17, 2007, from http://breastcrawl.org/pdf/breastcrawl.pdf
5. UNICEF/WHO. (2006, January) *Baby-Friendly Hospital Initiative, revised, updated and expanded for integrated care, Section 4, Hospital Self-Appraisal and Monitoring, Preliminary Version.* New York: UNICEF.
6. Emond, K. M., Zandoh, C., Quigley, M. A., Amenga-Etego, S., Owusu Agyei, S., & Kirkwood, B. (2006). Delayed breastfeeding initiation increases risk of neonatal mortality. *Pediatrics, 117*(3), e380–e386. Retrieved on September 17, 2007, from http://pediatrics.aappublications.org/cgi/content/abstract/117/3/e380
7. Ferber, S. G., & Makhoul, I. R. (2004). The effect of skin-to-skin contact (kangaroo care) shortly after birth on the neurobehavioral responses of the term newborn: A randomized, controlled trial. *Pediatrics, 113*(4), 858–865.
8. Ferber, S. G., & Makhoul, I. R. (2004). The effect of skin-to-skin contact (kangaroo care) shortly after birth on the neurobehavioral responses of the term newborn: A randomized, controlled trial. *Pediatrics, 113*(4), 863.
9. Carfoot, S., Williamson, P., & Dickson, R. (2005). A randomised controlled trial in the north of England examining the effects of skin-to-skin care on breast feeding. *Midwifery, 21*(1), 71–79.
10. Moore, E. R., Anderson, G. C., & Bergman, N. (2007). Early skin-to-skin contact for mothers and their healthy newborn infants. *Cochrane Database of Systematic Reviews,* (3), Art N:CD003519. DO1:10.1002/14651858.CD003519.pub2.
11. Widström, A. M., Ransjo-Arvidsön, A. B., Christensson, K., Matthiesen, A. S., Winberg, J., & Uvnäs-Moberg, K. (1987). Gastric suction in healthy newborn infants. *Acta paediatrica Scandinavica, 76,* 566–572.
12. Righard, L., & Alade, M. O. (1990). Effect of delivery room routines on success of first breast-feed. *Lancet, 336*(8723), 1105–1107.
13. American College of Obstetricians and Gynecologists. (2007). Breastfeeding: Maternal and infant aspects. Special report from ACOG. *ACOG Clinical Review, 12*(1 Suppl), 1S–16S.
14. American College of Obstetricians and Gynecologists. (2007). Breastfeeding: Maternal and infant aspects. Special report from ACOG. *ACOG Clinical Review, 12*(1 Suppl), 6S.
15. AAP Section on Breastfeeding. (2005). Breastfeeding and the use of human milk. *Pediatrics, 115,* 498–499.
16. Academy of Breastfeeding Medicine. (n.d.). *Protocol #5: Peripartum breastfeeding management for the healthy mother and infant at term.* Retrieved September 20, 2007, from http://bfmed.org/acefiles/protocol/peripartum.pdf, pp. 1–2.
17. AWHONN. (1999). *The role of the nurse in the promotion of breastfeeding: Clinical position statement.* Washington, DC. Available at http://awhonn.org/awhonn/content.do?name=05_HealthPolicyLegislation/5H_PositionStatements.htm.
18. World Health Organization. (2003). *Kangaroo mother care: A practical guide.* Geneva, Switzerland: Author. Retrieved February 2, 2008 at http://www.who.int/reproductive-health/publications/kmc/text.pdf

CHAPTER 5

Assessing and Supporting Breastfeeding Beyond the First Hour of Life

Key Steps in Supporting the Breastfeeding Couplet

The early postpartum period is when we see vertical and horizontal experiences of continuity of care come under the greatest challenge. Spelling out care practices explicitly in the policy document, and conducting practice audits and competency checks all contribute to assuring continuity of care.

Ideally, immediately after birth the mother and baby experience extended skin-to-skin contact, with the baby initiating the first feeding in the first hour or so of life (see Chapter 4 for more discussion of the first hour). Once these events have occurred, breastfeeding should be off to a good start.

However, breastfeeding assessment and support is needed throughout the postpartum stay and into the first weeks of life.

After the first self-attached feed, the mother and baby learn to work together and develop a collaborative feeding style.[1] It is the role of the mother to provide regular skin-to-skin contact, observe the baby for signs of feeding readiness, provide access to the breast, and hold the baby in a way that optimizes the baby's ability to attach well to the breast and to suckle effectively. Most mothers in North America have not grown up observing breastfeeding; thus, they instinctively mimic a holding position that they have seen when babies are bottle fed. This incorrect position often includes baby's head tucked in the inner crook of the mother's elbow, with the baby lying on its back, stomach facing up. This may be an ergonomically comfortable position for bottle-feeding, but it is not for breastfeeding. The baby must turn its head a quarter rotation toward the mother, and her breast must be made to turn to the baby. Turning both the baby's head and the mother's breast causes interference in the abilities for the baby to latch well and for the milk to flow freely.

Families also need help in deciphering the baby's feeding cues. Most adults associate crying with the baby's readiness for feeding. However, babies feed poorly in the crying state, which is the most distressed of all the infant states. Babies feed best in much earlier stages of alertness. Research indicates that newborn babies should be brought to the breast as soon as early feeding cues are seen, as any disruption (e.g., changing the diaper, getting a snack for the mother, etc.) may push the baby toward a more disorganized state.[2]

For this reason, staff responsible for the mother's care should be observing the baby's state and helping the family to identify and respond to indicators of feeding readiness (see Chapter 8 for more information about feeding cues). All families should learn these crucial cues, not just breastfeeding families! It is equally important that families who have chosen to formula-feed their babies learn how to prepare and feed formula.

Staff should also observe the breastfeeding mother's posture and infant positioning and offer suggestions as appropriate (see Box 5-1). Mothers need assistance in learning how to help babies achieve an appropriate grasp of the breast. Please see Box 5-2 for guidance on assisting the baby to latch optimally.

Mothers who are experiencing feeding discomfort and who have babies who are not receiving milk easily should be encouraged to make changes to the way the baby approaches and latches to the breast so that pain is relieved and milk flows freely. Staff delivering care at the postpartum bedside should have adequate knowledge and skills to address the common problems of the early postpartum period. In addition, lactation specialists[b] should be available to deal with more difficult problems and situations, including issues such as prematurity, craniofacial anomalies, ankyloglossia, and other physical challenges. Some have recommended a lactation specialist staffing ratio of roughly 1 full-time equivalent per 1000 births;[3] however, the actual number of specialist hours needed will be determined

---

[b] This would include lactation consultants certified by the International Board of Lactation Consultant Examiners, as well as other qualified professionals with specialized training and skill in lactation.

by the level of general staff competence in breastfeeding help, the rate of breastfeeding (facilities with higher breastfeeding rates will need more specialist time), the level of acuity of problems seen (e.g., number of high-risk deliveries, level of nursery care offered, etc.), and other expectations of the lactation staff (will they also teach classes, train staff, support mothers postdischarge, etc.?).

Box 5-1 **Breastfeeding Positions**

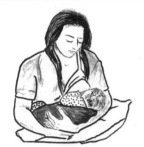

The cradle or Madonna posture:
- The mother sits in any posture that is comfortable.
- The baby lies on his or her side, facing the mother.
- The side of the baby's head and body rest on the mother's forearm of the arm next to the breast to be used.

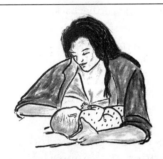

The cross-cradle posture:
This position is considered especially useful for the mother of a newborn or pre-term infant.
- The mother sits in any posture that is comfortable.
- The infant lies on his or her side, facing the mother.
- The side of the infant's body rests on the mother's forearm of the arm on the opposite side of the breast being used.
- The hand supports the baby's neck and shoulders in such a way that the baby can tilt his or her head.

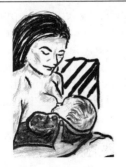

The football or clutch posture:
- The mother sits in any posture that is comfortable.
- The infant lies on his or her back, curled between the side of the mother's chest and her arm.
- The infant's upper body is supported by the mother's forearm.
- The mother's hand supports the infant's neck and shoulders.
- The infant's hips are flexed up along the chair back or other surface that the mother is leaning against.

/continues

Box 5-1 **Breastfeeding Positions (continued)**

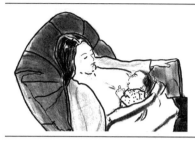

The semi-reclining posture:
- The mother sits in a comfortable, semi-reclining posture.
- The mother leans back and the baby lies against her body, usually prone.

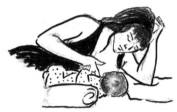

The side-lying posture:
- The mother lies on her side.
- The infant is placed on his or her side, lying chest to chest with mother.
- The mother's arm closest to the mattress or a rolled blanket supports the infant's back.

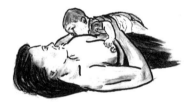

The Australian posture:
- The mother is "down-under," lying on her back.
- The baby is supported on her chest.
- This position is useful when the mother has a large milk supply or a powerful let-down as the baby has more ability to maneuver its head.

■ Expectations

Evaluation of the need for assistance and teaching begins at birth and continues throughout the hospital stay. A feeding should be evaluated during every nursing shift. In order to evaluate a feeding, the staff member needs to be in close proximity to the mother and baby, watching not only for details of the actual feeding, but also for the mother's knowledge of and response to infant cues, including hunger, fullness, desire for interaction, etc., as well as assessing the mother's and baby's comfort and watch-

ing for signs of milk transfer and need for further education and support. When staff have inadequate knowledge of appropriate feeding skills, and when they have a heavy workload, they may be tempted to evaluate breastfeeding by asking a mother closed questions such as "Is breastfeeding going OK?" This type of assessment is inadequate and can be misleading.

During the hospital stay, the breastfeeding woman needs to build confidence in her ability to breastfeed. Lack of maternal confidence has been identified as a significant risk factor for early cessation of breastfeeding by

Box 5-2   Achieving Comfortable and Effective Latch

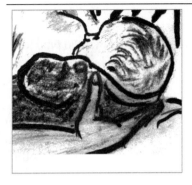

- The infant should be allowed the freedom he or she needs to achieve pain-free suckling with maximal milk transfer.
- The mother places the infant near the breast.
- Her hand supports the infant's shoulder at the base of the neck.
- There should be no pressure against the back of the infant's head from the mother's arm, hand, or from a pillow because the baby must be able to tilt his or her head.
- The infant's body is rotated toward the mother. This may be called "tummy to tummy" or "chest at the breast" or "chest to chest."

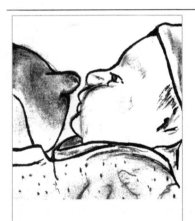

- The mother next moves the baby toward the breast, lining up the infant's nose at the nipple.
- The mother's breast should not be moved to the baby as this may distort the ducts and impede the natural flow of milk.
- Starting the feed with "nose to nipple" assists the infant to orient to the breast via a well-developed sense of smell and aligns the mouth at the breast when his or her head tilts back.

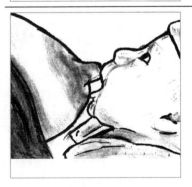

- The mother moves the infant 1 to 3 inches away from the nipple.
- As she moves the infant back toward the breast, he or she will gape, opening his or her mouth very wide as the head tilts back. If the infant fails to gape, the mother should repeat this maneuver.
- Consider an additional session of skin-to-skin holding to improve the infant's motor state organization for the infant who fails to gape or nurse.
- It is important for mothers not to push the nipple into the baby's mouth; this is unlikely to result in optimal positioning of the nipple or appropriate compression and release of the breast and nipple tissue during suckling.

numerous research teams.[4,5,6] The most helpful actions that can be provided by nursing staff are reflecting on the mother's growing skill at learning her baby's feeding cues and responding appropriately by assisting the baby in achieving a comfortable, productive attachment to the breast.

The Section on Breastfeeding of the American Academy of Pediatrics (AAP) recommends "Formal evaluation of breastfeeding, including observation of position, latch, and milk transfer, should be undertaken by trained caregivers at least twice daily and fully documented in the record during each day in the hospital after birth."[7]

To assure twice daily feeding assessment, it is recommended that a full feeding be observed as part of the task of the mother/baby nurse on each shift.

Any feeding problems identified during the hospital stay should be addressed and documented, complete with a discharge plan for further follow-up in the community. Research indicates that new mothers who abandon breastfeeding are most likely to do so in the early weeks of the baby's life, due to unresolved problems with latch, nipple discomfort, and milk supply concerns. It is crucial that problems encountered during the hospital stay are communicated to the mother's and baby's caregivers in the community, so that appropriate support and follow-up can be provided.

The AAP Section on Breastfeeding makes the following additional recommendations regarding feeding evaluation and problem identification:

Encouraging the mother to record the time and duration of each breastfeeding, as well as urine and stool output during the early days of breastfeeding in the hospital and the first weeks at home, helps to facilitate the evaluation process. Problems identified in the hospital should be addressed at that time, and a documented plan for management should be clearly communicated to both parents and to the medical home.[8]

The number of urinations daily in the newborn is an important indicator of kidney function; however, it does not reliably indicate *intake* as the baby is born with extra fluid store that is excreted over the first days after birth. For this reason, the number and color of *stools* produced is a better indicator of human milk intake. A general expectation is that the exclusively breastfed newborn will have one dark blackish-green meconium stool on the first day, followed by two greener stools on day 2, and three stools in the yellowish-green color range on day 3, with three or more loose, yellow stools expected daily every day after day 3 during the newborn period.

In addition to learning how to comfortably and effectively breastfeed, women should learn how to express their milk during their hospital stay. Manual or hand-expression is an essential and simple skill that should be taught to every new mother. Unless her infant is ill or premature, the mother does not need to learn to use a breast pump. Rather, the simple skill of manual milk expression should be taught. Manual expression is always available to the mother, regardless of electricity and availability of equipment, and can be used to release milk should she be separated from her baby. See Box 5-3 for more information.

After the birth of an early preterm baby, or of a baby with another condition that pre-

Box 5-3 Expression of Breastmilk

Hand Expression

Many women find that hand expression is easier and faster than using a mechanical breast pump. Another advantage to hand expression is that there is almost nothing to clean up or get contaminated (e.g., tubing, gaskets, etc.).

How we teach hand expression:

- Wash your hands.
- Have a clean container ready to collect the milk. The newer you are to hand expression, the wider the container should be. Start with a large, lightweight bowl for the first few expressions.
- Do light breast massage right down to your nipples. Give them a little stretch to get the hormones flowing.
- Place your thumb and index finger on your areola.

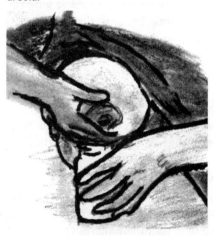

- Push back toward your chest wall, then compress your thumb and finger together gently. It is best if you do not slide your fingers on your skin. Some women like to use a rolling motion.
- Position the collecting container on a table if you are standing up, on your lap if you are sitting down. Try to aim the spray into the container.
- Repeat the push back and compress gently motion in the same place on your breast until the flow slows down.
- Move the finger and thumb to another spot and repeat.
- Switch to the other breast.
- Really proficient expressers can do both breasts simultaneously, but they usually need two bowls!

Breast Pumps

- Breast pumps should always be used and cleaned according to the manufacturer's instructions.
- There is no pump that is right for every mother and every situation. Some pumps are better for pump-dependent mothers and some are better for occasional use.
- Any pump can cause damage when used incorrectly.
- The U.S. Food and Drug Administration (FDA) maintains a database of pump complaints in the Manufacturer and User Facility Device Experience Database (MAUDE). See Appendix Y for more information. It is wise to check the database before considering pumps. Also, injuries related to breast pump use should be reported to the MAUDE site.
- There are several things to consider about operating a breast pump, such as whether it is powered by personal energy (hand or foot powered, for example) or powered by electricity, or whether it pumps one breast at a time or both together.
- Do not use parts from one company on another company's pumps.

cludes the initiation of breastfeeding in the early hours after birth, the mother should be assisted in initiating nipple stimulation and milk removal within six hours of giving birth. Stimulation of the breast within six hours of delivery has been correlated with greater milk supply in the ensuing weeks.[9] In the event that the mother and baby will be separated, maternity staff should endeavor to assist her in stimulating her milk supply, collecting her milk, and transporting it to the unit caring for her baby. In the event that the baby needs extended NICU care, NICU staff should support the mother in maintaining her milk supply and utilize expressed milk for the baby's nutrition as soon as possible.

Regarding the content of teaching and assessment during the postpartum stay, the Academy of Breastfeeding Medicine recommends the following:

> Breastfeeding mothers will be instructed about
> a. proper positioning and latch on;
> b. nutritive suckling and swallowing;
> c. milk production and release;
> d. frequency of feeding/feeding cues;
> e. expression of breast milk and use of a pump if indicated;
> f. how to assess if infant is adequately nourished; and
> g. reasons for contacting the clinician.

These skills will be taught to primiparous and multiparous women and reviewed before the mother goes home.[10]

■ Evidence

Consistent Advice

Numerous studies have identified the importance of consistent advice from all healthcare staff during the hospital stay. Women often receive inaccurate and inconsistent assistance from health staff, which they cite as a source of discontent with their postpartum care.[11] Kuan, Britto, Decolongon, Schoettker, Atherton, and Kotagal examined hospital factors associated with breastfeeding success and found that only 56% of women in the sample rated the support received in the hospital as good or very good.[12] Examining the experiences of new mothers and fathers, Dremsek, Göpfrich, Kurz, Bock, Benes, Philipp, and Sacher found that parents who reported receiving no breastfeeding support from maternity staff were less likely to initiate breastfeeding, while those who reported receiving little breastfeeding support experienced a higher rate of breastfeeding cessation in the first 3 months.[13] This research team also found that when parents reported that staff provided no information on breastfeeding, they were less likely to breastfeed, but when mothers received repeated breastfeeding information they were likely to breastfeed longer.

Building Maternal Confidence

What is the best way for staff to help mothers learn to breastfeed? There is sparse research evidence about the methods of various approaches. Some professionals use a hands-on approach to teaching, using their own hands to hold or adjust the position of the mother's breast and/or the baby. Research conducted with mothers who gave birth to preterm babies indicates that caution should be used in employing a hands-on approach to teaching. In a qualitative study, Weimers, Svensson, Dumas, Navér, and Wahlberg, V. report that most mothers in their population found hands-on techniques "unpleasant and not helpful mostly because it was unexpected and unexplained, [therefore] it would be important to either explain beforehand to mothers what type of physical approach could be attempted on their body or better, to avoid this type of approach completely."[14]

A small, qualitative study conducted by Hoddinott and Pill found that some women in their sample expressed discomfort with having their breasts handled by a health professional.[15] Breastfeeding is a learned skill; it may be learned best when the mother has the opportunity to repeat the process several times under her own control, coached appropriately by a knowledgeable caregiver.

In a cohort trial, a British hospital found that implementation of a hands-off teaching approach was associated with increases in exclusive breastfeeding at 2 weeks and 6 weeks of age, and a decrease in the number of mothers who perceived they had an inadequate milk supply.[16]

■ Common Barriers to Optimal Breastfeeding Assessment and Teaching and Strategies to Overcome Barriers

Inconsistent advice and teaching among staff is a major barrier to optimal breastfeeding teaching. It is best to implement staff breastfeeding training prior to tackling this barrier, as improved knowledge and skills development will assist in harmonizing advice and teaching given to mothers. As discussed in Chapter 2, it is crucial that staff training have practical, skills-oriented focus, so that staff members grow in competence and confidence in their abilities to assist mothers. Box 5-4 identifies the key role of competence. It is a mistake to assume that length of maternity care experience can predict breastfeeding knowledge and competence.

A helpful strategy for increasing consistency of breastfeeding care is to create a breastfeeding team, a group of individual staff members who have demonstrated skill and interest in breastfeeding. The team should observe one another working with breastfeeding couplets and establish a shared vision of what constitutes adequate and appropriate breastfeeding helping. The shared vision should be supported by the facility's breastfeeding policy and protocols, or the team should work with management to update and alter policies and procedures as needed.

Once the team has developed comfort with the shared vision of breastfeeding helping, the model of helping should be disseminated to the staff. This can be effectively achieved by having breastfeeding team members mentor individual staff members. Staff members begin by observing their breastfeeding mentor working with cases, and they eventually work under the supervision of the team member until the mentor can validate the competency of the staff member. All staff, regardless of length of experience in the field, can learn from observing each other working with families.

Some facilities use a breastfeeding assessment tool such as the Infant Breastfeeding Assessment Tool (IBFAT),[17] LATCH Assessment Tool (LATCH),[18] Latch-on

Assessment and corrective intervention Tool (LAT),[19] Mother-Baby Assessment for Breastfeeding (MBA),[20] or Systematic Assessment of the Infant at Breast (SAIB),[21] to provide a platform for identifying the parameters of breastfeeding assessment. Box 5-5 compares aspects of these tools.

In many U.S. health systems, financial constraints and staff shortages result in *overburdened workloads for healthcare workers*. Staff members who feel overwhelmed by the number of mother/baby couplets they must care for on each shift may not be able to give as much time and attention to the breastfeeding couplet as is needed. This situation can lead to burnout for the staff and to inadequate breastfeeding assessment, education, and support for the mother and baby.

One strategy for addressing this barrier is to create breastfeeding-helping circles that happen in a communal room on the maternity unit. This model, which is used in many hospitals around the world, allows a few staff members to work with several mother/baby couplets simultaneously. Mothers can be encouraged to gather in the solarium or other room on the unit (perhaps in the abandoned Level 1 nursery, once rooming-in is implemented—see Chapter 7) at certain times of the day for breastfeeding support. Staff members can facilitate dialogue between the mothers, answer questions, offer education and support, travel around the circle of mothers evaluating breastfeeding as it naturally occurs, offering practical suggestions on ways to im-

---

Box 5-4   The Power of Competence

We returned to a busy hospital (where more than 10,000 babies a year were born) a few weeks after training the postpartum nurses in skin-to-skin and latch-on skills. Marge, who had worked on the postpartum unit for more than 20 years, sought us out, took our hands in hers and tearfully told us that she could now help breastfeeding mothers. She went on to explain that in all her years of working with mothers and their newly born babies she never felt that she knew what to do. "When I got my assignments in the morning, I'd say to my manager: don't give me any breastfeeders," she said. "I knew that I couldn't help a mother with breastfeeding and with so many mothers breastfeeding today that was getting harder and harder to avoid getting the ones that breastfeed." She went on, "Now I can help! I put the baby skin

to skin and wait for the baby to latch on. I can even help the mother with her soreness by assessing the latch and helping her to correct it. I look forward to going to work again. I can't believe I could learn to do this." She laughed, "I guess you can teach an old dog new tricks!"

The Moral of the Story: Staff competence is important for improving breastfeeding outcomes, but also for staff well-being. Negative behavior regarding breastfeeding may be due to a staff member's lack of skill and confidence. Thus, training of all staff, regardless of years of experience in the field, should focus on assuring competence and confidence in the ability to assist mothers and babies with breastfeeding.

Box 5-5	**Characteristics of Commonly Used Breastfeeding Assessment and Documentation Tools**				
Characteristic	**LAT** Lactation Assessment Tool	**LATCH**	**IBFAT** Infant Breastfeeding Assessment Tool	**SAIB** Systematic Assessment of the Infant at Breast	**MBA** Mother-Baby Assessment
Scored by	Assessor	Mother or Nurse	Mother or Nurse	Nurse	Nurse
Time Frame	Progressive: beginning to ending	Static	Progressive: beginning to ending	Any point in the feeding	Progressive: beginning to ending
Scoring	Compares assessed findings with optimal	Expect increase in scores	Use mean of scores	Yes/No	Use best of scores
Assesses	Pre-feeding, latching and sucking dynamics	Latch-on Audible Swallowing Nipple Comfort Help Needed with positioning	Signaling Rooting Suckling	Alignment Areolar grasp Areolar compression Audible swallowing	Readiness Position Latch-on Milk Transfer Outcome

Modified from Biancuzzo, M. (2003). *Breastfeeding and the Newborn: Clinical Strategies for Nurses, Second Edition.* St. Louis: Mosby and Riordan J. M., Koehn M. J. *Journal of Obstetric, Gynecologic, and Neonatal Nursing, 26,* 183.

prove latch and positioning as needed, and triage problems and concerns. This model addresses many needs simultaneously, from providing contact with other mothers to allowing feeding assessment. It is preferable to models wherein the staff member or lactation specialist must spend an hour or more in an individual mother's room to see the baby attach, suckle, and feed. The model of helping one mother at a time is extremely time intensive, and cannot be scheduled, as babies need to be fed on their own internal schedule. It also helps women to learn breastfeeding by observing other mothers and babies breastfeeding. Mothers also meet one another, chat, and build networks, while staff members are efficiently helping multiple mother/baby pairs.

Another possible solution to the overburdened staff is to utilize volunteer breastfeeding peer counselors or to cross-train paraprofessionals such as nursing assistants in breastfeeding management. These individuals can visit with the breastfeeding women on the unit, sit with them through a feed to assess feeding skills, and determine if additional support is needed.

It may be best to wait to implement this step until routine skin-to-skin care in the first hours of life is firmly established as the facility norm. At this point, many breastfeeding infants will have experienced self-attachment, and should need less professional guidance in achieving appropriate latch-on, provided that the mother is supported in developing her collaborative feeding style. Once mothers and babies are off to a good start, staff should to spend less time remediating feeding problems caused by unnecessary mother/baby separation and lack of skin contact.

Some maternity staff members have a stated aversion to or *limited willingness to supporting breastfeeding families.* Care should be taken to identify those staff who lack confidence in their ability to assist or who have not had adequate training to feel competent with helping. In these cases, further training and support should be provided as needed. Working one on one with a breastfeeding mentor may be very helpful for individuals in this situation. Staff who lack competence or confidence in breastfeeding helping skills may shadow a mentor on the job, observing how the mentor assists several mother/baby couplets, and then gradually take over the counseling and helping with the guidance and support of the mentor. The mentor should be available in an ongoing way to the staff member, as a resource for second opinions and ad-

ditional assistance, and to take over lactation care for more difficult cases.

The job descriptions of staff delivering care to the mother and baby during the postpartum period should clearly indicate the breastfeeding helping expectations of the position. In the case where the apparent aversion to breastfeeding is not relieved by training and/or support, the unit manager must explore with the staff member the consequences of not performing to job requirements.

Resources

International Board of Lactation Consultant Examiners web site. Available at: www.iblce.org

References

1. Cadwell, K. (2007). Latching-on and suckling of the healthy term neonate: Breastfeeding assessment. *Journal of Midwifery and Women's Health, 52*(6), 638–642.
2. Anderson, G. C., Chiu, S-H., Morrison, B., Burkhammer, M., & Ludington-Hoe, S. (2004). Skin-to-skin for breastfeeding difficulties post-birth. In T. Field (Ed.), *Touch and massage in early child development.* New Brunswick, NJ: Johnson & Johnson, LLC pp.115–136
3. Riordan, J. (2005). *Breastfeeding and Human Lactation, Third Edition.* Sudbury, MA: Jones and Bartlett Publishers, p. 41.
4. Britton, J. R. (2007). Postpartum anxiety and breast feeding. *The Journal of Reproductive Medicine, 52*(8), 689–695.
5. Ertem, I. O., Votto, R. N., & Leventhal, M. D. (2001). The timing and predictors of the early termination of breastfeeding. *Pediatrics, 107*(3), 543–548.
6. Taveras, E. M., Capra, A. M., Braveman, P. A., Jensvold, N. G., Escobar, G. J., & Lieu, T. A. (2003). Clinician support and psychosocial risk factors associated with breastfeeding discontinuation. *Pediatrics, 112*(1 Pt 1), 108–115.
7. American Academy of Pediatrics, Section on Breastfeeding. (2005). Breastfeeding and the use of human milk. *Pediatrics, 115,* 498–499.

8. American Academy of Pediatrics, Section on Breastfeeding. (2005). Breastfeeding and the use of human milk. *Pediatrics,* 115, 499.

9. Furman, L., Minich, N., & Hack, M. (2002). Correlates of lactation in mothers of very low birth weight infants. *Pediatrics* 109(4):e57..

10. Chantry, C. J., Howard, C. R., & Philipp, B. L. (2007). ABM Clinical Protocol #7: Model Breastfeeding Policy. *Breastfeeding Medicine* 2(1), 51.

11. Rajan, L. (1993). The contribution of professional support, information and consistent correct advice to successful breast feeding. *Midwifery,* 9, 197–209.

12. Kuan, L. W., Britto, M., Decolongon, J., Schoettker, P. J., Atherton, H. D., & Kotagal, U. R. (1999). Health system factors contributing to breastfeeding success. *Pediatrics,* 104(3), e28.

13. Dremsek, P. A., Göpfrich, H., Kurz, H., Bock, W., Benes, K., Philipp, K. & Sacher, M. (2003). Stillberatung, Stillhäufigkeit und Stilldauer in einem Wiener Perinatalzentrum [Breast feeding support, incidence of breastfeeding and duration of breast feeding in a Vienna perinatal center]. *Wiener Medizinische Wochenschrift,* 153(11–12), 264–268. [Article in German].

14. Weimers, L., Svensson, K., Dumas, L., Navér, L., & Wahlberg, V. (2006). Hands-on approach during breastfeeding support in a neonatal intensive care unit: A qualitative study of Swedish mothers' experiences. *International Breastfeeding Journal, 1,* 20.

15. Hoddinott, P., & Pill, R. (2000). A qualitative study of women's views about how health professionals communicate about infant feeding. *Health Expectations,* 3(4), 224–233.

16. Ingram, J., Johnson, D., & Greenwood, R. (2002). Breastfeeding in Bristol: Teaching good positioning, and support from fathers and families. *Midwifery,* 18(2), 87–101.

17. Matthews, M. K. (1988). Developing an instrument to assess infant breastfeeding behavior in the early neonatal period. *Midwifery,* 4(4), 154.

18. Jensen, D., Wallace, S., & Kelsay, P. (1994). LATCH: A breastfeeding charting system and documentation tool. *Journal of Obstetric, Gynecologic and Neonatal Nursing,* 23(1), 27–32.

19. Healthy Children Project. (2000). *Latch-on assessment and corrective intervention tool (LAT).* East Sandwich, MA: Author.

20. Mulford, C. (1992). The mother-baby assessment (MBA): An "Apgar score" for breastfeeding. *Journal of Human Lactation,* 8, 79–82.

21. Shrago, L., & Bocar, D. (1990). The infant's contribution to breastfeeding. *Journal of Obstetric, Gynecologic and Neonatal Nursing,* 19(3), 209–215.

CHAPTER

6

Assuring Exclusive Breastfeeding

Exclusive breastfeeding means that the baby gets nothing else to eat except breastmilk. Although recommended by every credible authority for the first six months of life, it is rarely practiced in the United States and most other countries in the world. Why? Often mothers do not understand that the health benefits that they want for their baby come largely from exclusive breastfeeding. Also, they may not know what "exclusive" breastfeeding actually is. A researcher told us that the mothers in a study she was conducting who responded that they were exclusively breastfeeding were asked the follow-up question, "What else are you giving your baby to eat or drink?" Virtually every mother responded with cereal, formula, or another food. We can't expect mothers to achieve the goal of exclusive breastfeeding for six months unless they understand what it is.

■ Exclusive Breastfeeding: The Gold Standard of Infant Feeding

Healthy breastfeeding babies do not require routine supplementation with any food or drink other than human milk for the first 6 months, according to governmental, professional, and health organizations, including The United Nations Children's Fund (UNICEF), the World Health Organization (WHO), the American Academy of Pediatrics (AAP) Section on Breastfeeding, The American Academy of Family Physicians (AAFP), the Academy of Breastfeeding Medicine (ABM), and many others. After the first 6 months, appropriate complementary foods are added to the diet and breastfeeding should be continued for a year and beyond. According to an extensive systematic review:

> No deficits have been demonstrated in growth among infants from either de-

---

Box 6-1	**Medical Indications for Supplementing the Breastfed Baby (U.S. Committee for UNICEF)**

- Infants with severe dysmaturity
- Infants of very low birth weight
- Infants with inborn errors of metabolism
- Infants with acute water loss
- Infants whose mothers are severely ill
- Infants whose mothers require a medication that is contraindicated

Source: U.S. Committee for UNICEF & Wellstart International. Guidelines and Evaluation Criteria for Hospital/Birthing.

---

veloping or developed countries who are exclusively breastfed for 6 months or longer. Moreover, the mothers of such infants have more prolonged lactational amenorrhea and faster postpartum weight loss. Based on the results of this review, the World Health Assembly adopted a resolution to recommend exclusive breastfeeding for 6 months to its member countries.[1]

This finding has been upheld by a Cochrane Review.[2]

■ Expectations Regarding Exclusive Breastfeeding

Exclusive breastfeeding is defined as the baby receiving no supplementary feedings. Supplementary foods include manufactured breast milk substitutes such as formula, dextrose water, glucose water, juice, baby foods, and water. Exceptions are vitamins, minerals, and medications that have been prescribed for medical reasons. It is expected that the health system will not recommend routine supplementation of the breastfed newborn.

There may be individual cases where supplementation is medically indicated, but with optimal breastfeeding policies and practices, the incidence should be rare. The version of the WHO/UNICEF criteria, as developed by the U.S. Committee for UNICEF and Wellstart, for acceptable reasons for supplementation is found in Box 6-1. The draft version of the revised international criteria for supplementation is found in Box 6-2. One research study indicates that when supplements are given for medical reasons, there is an insignificant effect on breastfeeding outcomes.[3]

Box 6-2   UNICEF/WHO Acceptable Medical Reasons for Supplementation (DRAFT)

Exclusive breastfeeding is the norm. In a small number of situations there may be a medical indication for supplementing breastmilk or for not using breastmilk at all. It is useful to distinguish between:

- infants who cannot be fed at the breast but for whom breastmilk remains the food of choice;
- infants who may need other nutrition in addition to breastmilk;
- infants who should not receive breastmilk, or any other milk, including the usual
- breastmilk substitutes and need a specialised formula;
- infants for whom breastmilk is not available;
- maternal conditions that affect breastfeeding recommendations.

Infants who cannot be fed at the breast but for whom breastmilk remains the food of choice may include infants who are very weak, have sucking difficulties or oral abnormalities, or are separated from their mother who is providing expressed milk. These infants may be fed expressed milk by tube, cup, or spoon.

Infants who may need other nutrition in addition to breastmilk may include:

- very low birth weight or very preterm infants, i.e., those born less than 1500 g or 32 weeks gestational age;
- infants who are at risk of hypoglycaemia because of medical problems, when sufficient breastmilk is not immediately available; infants who are dehydrated or malnourished when breastmilk alone cannot restore the deficiencies.

These infants require an individualised feeding plan, and breastmilk should be used to the extent possible. Efforts should be made to sustain maternal milk production by encouraging expression of milk. Milk from tested milk donors may also be used. Hind milk is high in calories and particularly valuable for low birth weight infants.

Infants who should not receive breast milk, or any other milk, including the usual breastmilk substitutes may include infants with certain rare metabolic conditions such as galactosemia who may need feeding with a galactose free special formula or phenylketonuria where some breastfeeding may be possible, partly replaced with phenylalanine free formula.

Infants for whom breastmilk is not available may include when the mother had died, or is away from the baby and not able to provide expressed breastmilk. Breastfeeding by another woman may be possible; or the need for a breastmilk substitute may be only partial or temporary. There are a very few maternal medical conditions where breastfeeding is not recommended.

Maternal conditions that may affect breastfeeding recommendations include where the mother is physically weak, is taking medications, or has an infectious illness.

- A weak mother may be assisted to position her baby so her baby can breastfeed.
- A mother with a fever needs sufficient fluids.

Maternal medication
If mother is taking a small number of medications such as anti-metabolites, radioactive iodine, or some anti-thyroid medications, breastfeeding should stop during therapy.

/continues

Box 6-2 **UNICEF/WHO Acceptable Medical Reasons for Supplementation (DRAFT) (continued)**

Some medications may cause drowsiness or other side effects in the infant. Check medications with the WHO list, and where possible choose a medication that is safer and monitor the infant for side effects, while breastfeeding continues.

Maternal addiction

Even in situations of tobacco, alcohol and drug use, breastfeeding remains the feeding method of choice for the majority of infants. If mother is an intravenous drug user, breastfeeding is not indicated.

HIV-infected mothers

When replacement feeding is acceptable, feasible, affordable, sustainable and safe (AFASS), avoidance of all breastfeeding by HIV-infected mothers is recommended. Otherwise, exclusive breastfeeding is recommended during the first months of life, and should then be discontinued as soon as the specified conditions are met. Mixed feeding (breastfeeding and giving replacement feeds at the same time), is not recommended.

Other maternal infectious illnesses

- Breast abscess—feeding from the affected breast is not recommended but milk should be expressed from the breast. Feeding can be resumed once the abscess has been drained and the mother's treatment with antibiotics has commenced. Breastfeeding should continue on the unaffected breast.
- Herpes Simplex Virus Type I (HSV-1)— Women with herpes lesions on their breasts should refrain from breastfeeding until all active lesions on the breast have resolved.
- Varicella-zoster—Breastfeeding of a newborn infant is discouraged while the mother is infectious, but should be resumed as soon as the mother becomes non-infectious.
- Lyme disease—Breastfeeding may continue during mother's treatment.
- HTLV-I (Human T-cell leukaemia virus)— Breastfeeding is not encouraged if safe and feasible options (AFASS) for replacement feeding are available.

Even in situations where supplementation is necessary, the infant's nutrition should be continually assessed. Human milk should be used as much as possible. A clear policy regarding medical indications for supplementation and regular audits to assure adherence to the policy will reduce the risks of unwarranted supplementation. Often the breastfeeding committee appoints a subcommittee to review this issue and develop the supplementation section of the larger policy.

The *Ten Steps to Successful Breastfeeding* also expect that the birth facility will not accept free formula products, and will not give formula samples or other promotional items to breastfeeding families.

■ Effects of Supplementation on Specific Medical Conditions

Although optimal breastfeeding practices (such as early and frequent feeding, the elimination of routine supplements,[4] and effective latching with effective milk transfer) are recommended as a way to decrease the incidence of hyperbilirubinemia,[5,6] supplements of formula, sweetened water, and unsweetened water have also been used to prevent or cure newborn physiologic jaundice but have not been proven consistently effective. For example, numerous studies have failed to support the commonly held belief that supplementation with water or glucose water reduces hyperbilirubinemia of term, breastfed newborns.[7–10]

Healthy term infants who are breastfed on demand do not need sweetened water to prevent hypoglycemia[11] even if interfeed intervals are long.[12,13] Newborns who receive glucose water might lose more weight and stay in the hospital longer compared with infants who do not receive glucose water.[14] This may be because newborns are probably driven to feed by thirst rather than hunger and sweetened or unsweetened water lessens interest in breastfeeding.[15]

■ Barriers to Exclusive Breastfeeding and Strategies to Overcome Them

Common Nonmedical Reasons for Supplementation of the Newborn

There may be other hospital practices related to routine supplementation without medical indications.[16,17] *Separation of mothers and babies*[18] and the staff believing that the baby is hungry or thirsty[19] are both related to increased use of supplements. Mothers may also give their baby supplements in the hospital because of a mistaken belief that their milk is insufficient.[20,21]

Starting formula supplementation after hospital discharge because of *concern about the adequacy of mother's milk* supply is also significantly related to early cessation of breastfeeding.[22] Other factors related to supplementation include adolescent mother, fewer than six prenatal visits, using a pacifier within the first month, poor latch-on,[23] maternal smoking,[24] recent immigration,[25] planning to return to work outside the home,[26] and a high maternal anxiety trait.[27]

The Effect of Early Supplementation on the Baby

Although questions remain as to the effect on breastfeeding outcome of a brief exposure in the maternity setting to sweetened and unsweetened water, formula, or other liquids on the success and duration of breastfeeding,[28–35] there are indications that exposure to cow's-milk-based formula before 9 days may be related an increased risk of the baby later developing Type 1 diabetes (T1DM).[36] The same result has been seen with shorter durations of breastfeeding[37] and early introduction of cereal.[38]

Even a few feedings of formula may result in the development of cow's-milk intolerance or cow's-milk allergy, which becomes symptomatic in later infancy,[39,40] especially in babies whose parents had obvious allergic symptoms.

Supplements also increase the risk of diarrhea, meningitis, and neonatal sepsis, particularly when combined with poor hygiene[41–44] and when powdered infant formula is used.[45,46] Powdered infant formula is not sterile and may contain pathogenic organisms. In addition, milk products are excellent media for bacterial proliferation according to a commentary of the Committee on Nutrition of the European Society of Paediatric Gastroenterology, Hepatology and Nutrition (ESPGHAN). Of particular concern is the multiplication of

Enterobacter sakazakii in prepared formula feeds, which can cause sepsis.[47] Even in conditions with better hygiene, exclusively breastfed babies have fewer illnesses than those that are supplemented.[48,49] It is crucial that parents who are formula-feeding learn safe techniques for preparing and storing formula. Safe food handling techniques are essential to reduce risk of contamination and illness.

Contraindications to Breastfeeding

Of course, some women will choose to not breastfeed and other women should not breastfeed. The CDC's list of women who absolutely should not breastfeed is published on its web site and is revised as information changes. Box 6-3 lists the reasons that were current at the date of this book's publication. However, mothers and healthcare providers often have *misconceptions about conditions and medications that may contraindicate breastfeeding.* We've been told by a medical care provider that a mother should not breastfeed because she has received some benign medication such as ibuprofen, or that she should cease breastfeeding while she has the flu (both untrue). In general, care providers are poorly educated about the safety of combining breastfeeding with medications and other medical conditions. If they are not aware of resources such as those appearing at the end of this chapter, they may advise a mother incorrectly that it is best to stop breastfeeding.

Surprisingly few medications, conditions, or procedures require even a brief hiatus from feeding the baby mother's milk. For specific recommendations, resources specific to lactation are available and are listed in the resource sections at the end of this chapter.

Box 6-3 **The CDC's List of Women Who Should Not Breastfeed**

At the time of publication of this book, the Centers for Disease Control and Prevention advises women in the United States not to breastfeed if one or more of the following conditions exists:

- The infant has been diagnosed with galactosemia
- The breastfeeding mother:
  - Has been infected with the human immunodeficiency virus (HIV)
  - Is taking antiretroviral medications
  - Has untreated, active tuberculosisIs infected with human T-cell lymphotropic virus (HTLV), Type I or Type II
  - Is using or are dependent upon an illicit drug
  - Is taking prescribed cancer chemotherapy agents, such as antimetabolites that interfere with DNA replication and cell division
  - Is undergoing radiation therapies; however, such nuclear medicine therapies require only a temporary interruption in breastfeeding

Source: Centers for Disease Control and Prevention. (2007). *When Should a Woman Avoid Breastfeeding?* Atlanta, GA: Author. Retrieved on 02/14/07 at http://www.cdc.gov/breastfeeding/disease/contraindicators.htm.

Marketing Formula to Parents—An Ethical and Commercial Conundrum

Formula is widely available in our birth settings; the omnipresence of formula samples seems to cause many parents and care providers to resort to *thinking of formula as a solution for all breastfeeding problems*. The omnipresence of formula is a violation of the International Code of Marketing of Breastmilk Substitutes (the Code). Parents are protected from formula marketing by the Code and subsequent World Health Assembly (WHA) resolutions. National and transnational companies continue to market breast milk substitutes in violation of the Code, including providing free samples, items bearing formula company names or logos, coupons for formula, etc. to new parents through hospital distribution. In addition, the WHO/UNICEF Baby-Friendly hospital standards stipulate that there is to be no promotion for infant foods or drinks other than breast milk by a hospital practicing the *Ten Steps to Successful Breastfeeding*.[50]

Hospitals give mothers discharge packs or gift bags containing coupons and other advertisements. This has been done in the past even without the knowledge of the medical staff.[51] Some of these bags include free samples of formula, feeding bottles, and nipples. Mothers who receive free formula samples at discharge may be more likely to use formula (and in some studies also start solid foods earlier) than mothers who do not receive samples regardless of infant feeding intentions at admission.[52–54]

There was no significant difference in research studies between mothers who received discharge packs with free formula samples and mothers who were given breast pumps in their gift bags.[55,56] Not all women will need breast pumps. The first time a new mother uses a pump, it is rare for her to have a measurable yield of milk. This is due to the viscous nature of her milk as well as the fact that it takes time for women to learn to let-down their milk to a mechanical device. The mother is rarely aware of these factors, and thus may mistakenly believe that the limited amount of milk expressed indicates a problem with her milk supply. This is another reason why hand expression of milk should be the focus of education during the hospital stay. Some hospitals give mothers a small plastic spoon as their collection vessel. The limited size of the container helps to set a reasonable expectation of the yield. Using breast pumps as an incentive has not been shown to be an effective breastfeeding promotion strategy.

Gift packs from formula companies are not limited in their distribution through the hospital. Companies may promote their products to the general public through the media or selectively through targeted health professionals and clinics. Women randomly selected to receive either a formula company gift pack or a specially designed breastfeeding education pack at their first prenatal visit with an obstetrician were followed through the postpartum period to determine breastfeeding outcomes. Exposure to the formula company material significantly increased breastfeeding cessation before hospital discharge and in the first 2 weeks.[57] The brand of formula used in the hospital influences a mother to purchase the same brand after discharge.[58]

Nowhere else in the healthcare system are commercial gift packs distributed to patients at discharge. In return for giving the discharge bag to new mothers, the health system receives kickbacks from the company for the right to advertise to patients. This kind of arrangement is at odds with modern healthcare ethics. Hospitals and health systems across the United States have recognized the disadvantages of distributing free formula and the accompanying advertising to new families and created new bags to distribute. These bags often have the hospital's logo and are filled with educational materials about lead paint screening, immunizations, local mommy and baby classes, breastfeeding support groups, etc.

Hospital leaders have also come to realize the ethical problems inherent in their relationships with formula and other companies and have put into place strict vendor policies that limit the amount of physical access the sales representatives and company educators are allowed to have in the facility as well as restricting the access of vendors to patients and staff. Vendors are also prohibited from giving gifts above a certain value, usually a small amount ($5 or less) to staff or members of the management team. For additional points in the Code relevant to hospitals and birth centers, please see Box 6-4.

When a hospital or birth center decides to purchase formula and other feeding equipment, *concern arises about the amount of money that will need to be spent.* See Box 6-5. Staff at one hospital have shared their experience of moving to a more businesslike arrangement with a formula company.[59]

In the event that the birth facility does not purchase formula, it is our strong recommendation is that the birth facility consider delaying the process of purchase of formula until the remaining practice steps of the *Ten Steps to Successful Breastfeeding* are in place. At that point, the majority of health system practices that contribute to unnecessary formula supplementation should be corrected, the exclusive breastfeeding rate should be greatly increased, and the volume of formula that the facility will need to purchase will be decreased.

Box 6-4 | **Articles 6 and 7 of the International Code of Marketing of Healthcare Systems**

Article 6. Healthcare systems

6.1 The health authorities in Member States should take appropriate measures to encourage and protect breastfeeding and promote the principles of this Code, and should give appropriate information and advice to health workers in regard to their responsibilities, including the information specified in Article 4.2.

6.2 No facility of a healthcare system should be used for the purpose of promoting infant formula or other products within the scope of this Code. This Code does not, however, preclude the dissemination of information to health professionals as provided in Article 7.2.

6.3 Facilities of healthcare systems should not be used for the display of products within the scope of this Code, for placards or posters concerning such products, or for the distribution of material provided by a manufacturer or distributor other than that specified in Article 4.

6.4 The use by the healthcare system of "professional service representatives," "mothercraft nurses" or similar personnel, provided or paid for by manufacturers or distributors, should not be permitted.

/continues

<table><tr><td>**Box 6-4**</td><td>**Articles 6 and 7 of the International Code of Marketing of Healthcare Systems (continued)**</td></tr></table>

6.5 Feeding with infant formula, whether manufactured or home prepared, should be demonstrated only by health workers, or other community workers if necessary; and only to the mothers or family members who need to use it; and the information given should include a clear explanation of the hazards of improper use.

6.6 Donations or low-price sales to institutions or organisations of supplies of infant formula or other products within the scope of this Code, whether for use in the institutions or for distribution outside them, may be made. Such supplies should only be used or distributed for infants who have to be fed on breastmilk substitutes. If these supplies are distributed for use outside the institutions, this should be done only by the institutions or organisations concerned. Such donations or low-price sales should not be used by manufacturers or distributors as a sales inducement.

6.7 Where donated supplies of infant formula or other products within the scope of this Code are distributed outside an institution, the institution or organisation should take steps to ensure that supplies can be continued as long as the infants concerned need them. Donors, as well as institutions or organisations concerned, should bear in mind this responsibility.

6.8 Equipment and materials, in addition to those referred to in Article 4.3, donated to a healthcare system may bear a company's name or logo, but should not refer to any proprietary product within the scope of this Code.

Article 7. Health workers

7.1 Health workers should encourage and protect breastfeeding; and those who are concerned in particular with maternal and infant nutrition should make themselves familiar with their responsibilities under this Code, including the information specified in Article 4.2.

7.2 Information provided by manufacturers and distributors to health professionals regarding products within the scope of this Code should be restricted to scientific and factual matters, and such information should not imply or create a belief that bottle feeding is equivalent or superior to breastfeeding. It should also include the information specified in Article 4.2.

7.3 No financial or material inducements to promote products within the scope of this Code should be offered by manufacturers or distributors to health workers or members of their families, nor should these be accepted by health workers or members of their families.

7.4 Samples of infant formula or other products within the scope of this Code, or of equipment or utensils for their preparation or use, should not be provided to health workers except when necessary for the purpose of professional evaluation or research at the institutional level. Health workers should not give samples of infant formula to pregnant women, mothers of infants and young children, or members of their families.

7.5 Manufacturers and distributors of products within the scope of this Code should disclose to the institution to which a recipient health worker is affiliated any contribution made to him or on his behalf for fellowships, study tours, research grants, attendance at professional conferences, or the like. Similar disclosures should be made by the recipient.

Source: World Health Organization (1981). *International Code of Marketing of Breast-milk Substitutes.* Geneva, Switzerland: Author.

Box 6-5 Buying Formula for Hospital or Birth Center Use

It is recommended that before estimating how much it will cost to buy formula, one should conduct an audit in order to be sure that all of the policies and practices that support breastfeeding prior to discharge are in place, including the following:

- Prenatal education
- Breastfeeding policy
- Staff training
- Early skin-to-skin contact
- Help with breastfeeding
- Twenty-four hour rooming-in
- No restrictions on breastfeeding frequency or duration of feedings
- Collection and storage of breast milk
- Supplement use for medical indications only
- Noncommercial and accurate patient education materials
- No routine distribution of pacifiers, bottles, or bottle nipples

The next step is to restrict formula use to babies whose mothers have chosen to feed formula and to breastfed babies who have medical indications for formula supplementation. A problem that hospitals have noticed is that since staff members perceive formula to be free, it's given away liberally.

One way that hospitals have been able to successfully estimate the amount of formula that is actually needed is to lock up the formula and require formula withdrawn to be logged out, noting the formula batch number (in case there is a recall), date and time, patient and staff members' names or identification numbers, and reason for use. Another way hospitals manage formula use is via a medication distribution system such as Pyxis. This will help to restrict formula usage, as well as provide information about what additional education and skill areas need to be advanced among staff.

After collecting usage data for a period of time, hospital staff should put a bid out to vendors, including large chain pharmacies or food wholesalers to determine the fair market price of formula.

Resources

Academy of Breastfeeding Medicine. (2002). *Clinical Protocol #3: ABM clinical protocol number 3—Hospital guidelines for the use of supplementary feedings in the healthy term breastfed neonate.* New Rochelle, NY: Author.

American Academy of Pediatrics. (1997). Breastfeeding and the use of human milk. *Pediatrics, 100*(6),1035–1039.

American Academy of Pediatrics. (2004). Management of hyperbilirubinemia in the newborn infant 35 or more weeks of gestation. *Pediatrics, 114*(1), 297–316.

Ban the Bags Campaign. www.banthebags.org.

Donnelly, A., Snowden, H. M., Renfrew, M. J., & Woolridge, M. W. (2000). Commercial hospital discharge packs for breastfeeding women. *Cochrane Database of Systematic Reviews.* (2):CD002075.

Walker, M. (2001, 2007) *Selling out mothers and babies: Marketing of breast milk substitutes in the USA.* Weston, MA: National Alliance for Breastfeeding Advocacy, Research, Education and Legal Branch. Find information about the latest edition at: naba-breastfeeding.org/resources.htm

Wight, N., Marinelli, K. A., Academy of Breastfeeding Medicine Protocol Committee. (2006). *ABM clinical protocol #1: Guidelines for glucose monitoring and treatment of hypoglycemia in breastfed neonates.* Breastfeeding Medicine, 1(3), 178–184.

World Health Organization. (1997). *Hypoglycemia of the newborn: Review of the literature.* Geneva, Switzerland: Author.

Resources for Medications and Breastfeeding

AAP Committee on Drugs. (2001). The transfer of drugs and other chemicals into human milk. *Pediatrics, 108,* 776–789. Available at www.aappolicy.aappublications.org/cgi/content/full/pediatrics.

Drugs and Lactation Database (LactMed). Bethesda, MD: National Library of Medicine. Available at: http://toxnet.nlm.nih.gov/cgi-bin/sis/htmlgen?LACTHale, T. *Medications and mother's milk.* Available at: http://www.ibreastfeeding.com/Lawrence, R. A., Lawrence, R. M. (2005) *Breastfeeding: A guide for the medical profession,* 5th Edition St. Louis, MO: Mosby. [Be sure to get the latest edition.]

World Health Organization. (1981). *International Code of Marketing of Breast-milk Substitutes.* Geneva, Switzerland: Author. Available at www.who.int/nutrition/publications/code_english.pdf. Subsequent World Health Assembly resolutions are accessible at: http://www.ibfan.org/english/resource/who/whares3332.html.

References

1. Kramer, M. S., & Kakuma, R. (2004). The optimal duration of exclusive breastfeeding: A systematic review. *Advances in Experimental Medicine and Biology, 554,* 63.
2. Kramer, M. S., & Kakuma, R. (2002). Optimal duration of exclusive breastfeeding. *Cochrane Database of Systematic Reviews.* (1):CD003517.
3. Blomquist, H. K., Jonsbo, F., Sereniuius, F., & Persson, L. A. (1994). Supplementary feeding in the maternity ward shortens the duration of breast feeding. *Acta Paediatrica,* 83(11), 1122–1126.
4. Nylander, G., Lindemann, R., Helsing, E., & Bendvold, E. (1991). Unsupplemented breastfeeding in the maternity ward. Positive long-term effects. *Acta Obstetrica Gynecologica Scandinavica,* 70, 205–209.
5. Semmekrot, B. A., de Vries, M. C., Gerrits, G. P., & van Wieringen, P. M. (2004). Optimale borstvoeding ter preventie van hyperbilirubinemie bij gezonde, voldragen pasgeborenen [Optimal breastfeeding to prevent hyperbilirubinaemia in healthy, term newborns]. *Nederlands Tijdschrift Voor Geneeskunde,* 148(41), 2016–2019. [Article in Dutch]
6. Niestijl, A. L., & Sauer, P. J. (2003). Breastfeeding during the first few days after birth: Sometimes insufficient. *Nederlands Tijdschrift Voor Geneeskunde,* 147(49), 2405–2407.
7. Verronen, P., Visakorpi, J. K., Lammi, A., Saarikoski, S., & Taminen, T. (1980). Promotion of breast feeding: Effect on neonates of change of feeding routine at a maternity unit. *Acta Paediatrica Scandinavica,* 69, 279–282.
8. de Carvalho, M., Hall, M., & Harvey, D. (1981). Effects of water supplementation on physiological jaundice in breast-fed babies. *Archives of Disease in Childhood,* 56(7), 568–569.
9. Nicoll, A., Ginsburg, R., & Tripp, J. H. (1982). Supplementary feeding and jaundice in newborns. *Acta Paediatrica Scandinavica,* 71, 759–761.
10. Nylander, G., Lindemann, R., Helsing, E., & Bendvold, E. (1991). Unsupplemented breastfeeding in the maternity ward. Positive long-term effects. *Acta Obstetrica Gynecologica Scandinavica,* 70, 205–209.
11. de Carvalho, M., Hall, M., & Harvey, D. (1981). Effects of water supplementation on physiological jaundice in breast-fed babies. *Archives of Disease in Childhood,* 56(7), 568–569.
12. Williams, A. F. (1997). Hypoglycaemia of the newborn: a review. *Bulletin of the World Health Organization,* 75(3), 261–290.
13. Martin-Calama, J., Buñuel, J., Valero, M. T., Labay, M., Lasarte, J. J., Valle, F., et al. (1997). The effect of feeding glucose water to breastfeeding newborns on weight, body temperature, blood glucose, and breastfeeding duration. *Journal of Human Lactation,* 13(3), 209–213.
14. Glover, J., & Sandilands, M. (1990). Supplementation of breastfeeding infants and weight loss in hospital. *Journal of Human Lactation,* 6(4), 163–166.
15. Kuhr, M., & Paneth, N. (1982). Feeding practices and early neonatal jaundice. *Journal of Pediatric Gastroenterology and Nutrition,* 1(4), 485–488.
16. Alikasifo lu, M., Erginoz, E., Gur, E. T., Baltas, Z., Beker, B., & Arvas, A. (2001). Factors influencing the duration of exclusive breastfeeding in a group of Turkish women. *Journal of Human Lactation,* 17(3), 220–226.
17. Martin-Calama, J., Buñuel, J., Valero, M. T., Labay, M., Lasarte, J. J., Valle, F., et al. (1997). The effect of feeding glucose water to breastfeeding newborns on weight, body temperature, blood glucose, and breastfeeding duration. *Journal of Human Lactation,* 13(3), 209–213.

18. Faldella, G., Di Comite, A., Marchiani, E., Govoni, M., Salvioli, G. P. (1999). Breastfeeding duration and current neonatal feeding practices in Emilia Romagna, Italy. *Acta Paediatrica Supplement, 88*(430), 23–26.

19. Akuse, R. M., & Obinya, E. A. (2002). Why health care workers give prelacteal feeds. *European Journal of Clinical Nutrition, 56*(8), 729–734.

20. Aghaji, M. N. (2002). Exclusive breast-feeding practice and associated factors in Enugu, Nigeria. *West African Journal of Medicine, 21*(1), 66–69.

21. Hossain, M. M., Radwan, M. M., Arafa, S. A., Habib, M., & DuPont, H. L. (1991). Prelacteal infant feeding practices in rural Egypt. *Journal of Tropical Pediatrics, 38*(6), 317–322.

22. Pérez-Escamilla, R., Seguar-Millan, S., Pollitt, E., & Dewey, K. G. (1993). Determinants of lactation performance across time in an urban population from Mexico. *Social Science and Medicine, 37*(8), 1069–1078.

23. Santo, L. C., de Oliveira, L. D., & Giugliani, E. R. (2007, September). Factors associated with low incidence of exclusive breastfeeding for the first 6 months. *Birth, 34*(3), 212–219.

24. Butler, S., Williams, M., Tukuitonga, C., & Paterson, J. (2004). Factors associated with not breastfeeding exclusively among mothers of a cohort of Pacific infants in New Zealand. *The New Zealand Medical Journal, 117*(1195), U908.

25. Romero-Gwynn, E. (1989). Breast-feeding pattern among Indochinese immigrants in northern California. *American Journal of Diseases of Children, 143*(7), 804–808.

26. Chezem, J., Friesen, C., Montgomery, P., Fortman, R., & Clark, H. (1998). Lactation duration: Influences of human milk replacements and formula samples on women planning postpartum employment. *Journal of Obstetric, Gynecologic, and Neonatal Nursing, 27*(6), 646–651.

27. Gagnon, A. J., Leduc, G., Waghorn, K., Yang, H., & Platt, R. W. (2005). In-hospital supplementation of healthy breastfeeding newborns. *Journal of Human Lactation, 21*(4), 397–405.

28. Szajewska, H., Horvath, A., Koletzko, B., & Kalisz, M. (2006). Effects of brief exposure to water, breastmilk substitutes, or other liquids on the success and duration of breastfeeding: A systematic review. *Acta Paediatrica, 95*(2), 145–152.

29. Pérez-Escamilla, R., Maulén-Radovan, I., & Dewey, K. G. (1996). The association between cesarean delivery and breastfeeding outcomes among Mexican women. *American Journal of Public Health, 86*(6), 832–836.

30. Gray-Donald, K., Kramer, M. S., Munday, S., & Leduc, D. G. (1985). Effect of formula supplementation in the hospital on the duration of breastfeeding: A controlled clinical trial. *Pediatrics, 75*(3), 514–518.

31. Kind, C., Schubiger, G., Schwarz, U., & Tönz, O. (2000). Provision of supplementary fluids to breast fed infants and later breast feeding success. *Advances in Experimental Medicine and Biology, 478,* 347–354.

32. Kurinij, N., Axelson, M. L., Forman, M. R., & Weingold, A. B. (1984). Predicting duration of breastfeeding in a group of urban primiparae. *Ecology of Food and Nutrition, 15,* 281–291.

33. Giovannini, M., Riva, E., Banderali, G., Salvioni, M., Radaelli, G., & Agostoni, C. (2005). Exclusive versus predominant breastfeeding in Italian maternity wards and feeding practices through the first year of life. *Journal of Human Lactation, 21*(3), 259–265.

34. Feinstein, J. M., Berkelhamer, J. E., Gruszka, M. E., Wong, C. A., & Carey, A. E. (1986). Factors related to early termination of breast-feeding in an urban population. *Pediatrics, 78*(2), 210–215.

35. Martens, P. J. (2000). Does breastfeeding education affect nursing staff beliefs, exclusive breastfeeding rates, and Baby-Friendly Hospital Initiative compliance? The experience of a small, rural Canadian hospital. *Journal of Human Lactation, 16*(4), 309–318.

36. Gimeno, S. G., & de Souza, J. M. (1997, August). IDDM and milk consumption: A case-control study in São Paulo, Brazil. *Diabetes Care, 20*(8), 1256–1260.

37. Sadauskaite-Kuehne, V., Ludvigsson, J., Padaiga, Z., Jasinskiene, E., & Samuelsson, U. (2004, March–April). Longer breastfeeding is an independent protective factor against development of type 1 diabetes mellitus in childhood. *Diabetes/Metabolism Research and Reviews, 20*(2), 150–157.

38. Norris, J. M., Barriga, K., Klingensmith, G., Hoffman, M., Eisenbarth, G. S., Erlich, H. A., et al. (2003, October 1). Timing of initial cereal exposure in infancy and risk of islet autoimmunity. *Journal of the American Medical Association, 290*(13), 1713–1720.

39. Høst, A. (1991). Importance of the first meal on the development of cow's milk allergy and intolerance. *Allergy Proceedings, 12*(4), 227–232.

40. Saarinen, K. M., Juntunen-Backman, K., Järvenpää, A. L., Kuitunen, P., Lope, L., Renlund, M., et al. (1999). Supplementary feeding in maternity hospitals and the risk of cow's milk allergy: A prospective study of 6209 infants. *The Journal of Allergy and Clinical Immunology, 104*(2 Pt 1), 457–461.

41. Victora, C. G., Smith, P. G., Vaughan, J. P., Nobre, L. C., Lombardi, C., Teixeira, A. M., et al. (1987). Evidence for the protection by breast-feeding against infant deaths from infectious diseases in Brazil. *Lancet, 2*(8554), 319–322.

42. de Zoysa, I., Rea, M., & Martines, J. (1991). Why promote breastfeeding in diarrhoeal disease control programmes? *Health Policy and Planning, 6*(4), 371–379.

43. Ashraf, R. N., Jalil, F., Zaman, S., Karlberg, J., Khan, S. R., Linblad, B. S., et al. (1991). Breast feeding and protection against neonatal sepsis in a high risk population. *Archives of Disease in Childhood, 66*(4), 488–490.

44. Avoa, A., & Fischer, P. R. (1990). The influence of perinatal instruction about breast-feeding on neonatal weight loss. *Pediatrics, 86*(2), 313–315.

45. MMWR Morbidity and Mortality Weekly Report. (2002). *Enterobacter sakazakii* infection associated with the use of powdered infant formula–Tennessee, 2001. *MMWR Morbidity and Mortality Weekly Report, 51*(14), 297–300.

46. Block, C., Peleg, O., Minster, N., Bar-Oz, B., Simhon, A., Arad, I., et al. (2002). Cluster of neonatal infections in Jerusalem due to unusual biochemical variant of *Enterobacter sakazawii*. *European Journal of Clinical Microbiology and Infectious Diseases, 21*(8), 613–616.

47. Agostoni, C., Axelsson, I., Goulet, O., Koletzko, B., Michaelsen, K. F., Puntis, J. W., et al. (2004). Preparation and handling of powdered infant formula: A commentary by the ESPGHAN committee on nutrition. *Journal of Pediatric Gastroenterology and Nutrition, 39*(4), 320–322.

48. Howie, P. W. (1990). Protective effect of breast feeding against infection. *British Medical Journal, 300*, 11–16.

49. Raisler, J., Alexander, C., & O'Campo, P. (1999, January). Breast-feeding and infant illness: A dose-response relationship? *American Journal of Public Health, 89*(1), 25–30.

50. Merewood, A., & Philipp, B. L. (2000). Becoming baby-friendly: Overcoming the issue of accepting free formula. *Journal of Human Lactation, 16*(4), 279–282.

51. Hayden, G. F., Noawcek, G. A., Koch, W., & Kattwinkel, J. (1987). Providing free samples of baby items to newly delivered parents. An unintentional endorsement? *Clinical Pediatrics, 26*(3), 111–115.

52. Margen, S., Melnick, V., Neuhauser, L., & Rios, E. (1991). *Infant feeding in Mexico. A study of health facility and mothers' practices in three regions.* Washington, DC: Nestlé Infant Formula Audit Commission.

53. Pérez-Escamilla, R., Pollitt, E., Lönnerdal, B., Dewey, K. G. (1994). Infant feeding policies in maternity wards and their effect on breast-feeding success: An analytical overview. *American Journal of Public Health, 84*(1), 89–97.

54. Donnelly, A., Snowden, H. M., Renfrew, M. J., & Woolridge, M. W. (2000). Commercial discharge packs for breastfeeding women. *Cochrane Database of Systematic Reviews*, (2):CD0020745.

55. Bliss, M. C., Wilkie, J., Acredolo, C., Berman, S., & Tebb, K. P. (1997). The effect of discharge pack formula and breast pumps on breastfeeding duration and choice of infant feeding method. *Birth, 24*(2), 90–97.

56. Dungy, C. I., Losch, M. E., Russell, D., Romitti, P., & Dusdieker, L. B. (1997). Hospital infant formula discharge packages. Do they affect the duration of breast-feeding? *Archives of Pediatric and Adolescent Medicine, 151*(7), 724–729.

57. Howard, C. R., Howard, F., Lawrence, R., Andresen, E., DeBlieck, E., & Weitzmana, M. (2000). Office prenatal formula advertising and its effect on breastfeeding patterns. *Obstetrics and Gynecology, 95*(2), 269–303.

58. Reiff, M. I., & Essock-Vitale, S. M. (1985). Hospital influences on early infant-feeding practices. *Pediatrics, 76*, 872–879.

59. Merewood, A., & Philipp, B. L. (2000). Becoming baby-friendly: Overcoming the issue of accepting free formula. *Journal of Human Lactation, 16*, 272–282.

Ten Steps to Successful Breastfeeding
A Joint WHO/UNICEF Statement[a]

Every facility providing maternity services and care for newborn infants should:

1. Have a written breastfeeding policy that is routinely communicated to all healthcare staff.
2. Train all healthcare staff in skills necessary to implement this policy.
3. Inform all pregnant women about the benefits and management of breastfeeding.
4. Help mothers initiate breastfeeding within a half-hour of birth. (US, one hour)
5. Show mothers how to breastfeed, and how to maintain lactation even if they should be separated from their infants.
6. Give newborn infants no food or drink other than breastmilk unless medically indicated.
7. **Practice rooming in—allow mothers and infants to remain together—24 hours a day.**
8. Encourage breastfeeding on demand.
9. Give no artificial teats (US, nipples) or pacifiers (also called dummies or soothers) to breastfeeding infants.
10. Foster the establishment of breastfeeding support groups and refer mothers to them on discharge from the hospital or clinic.

[a] World Health Organization. (1989). *Protecting, promoting and supporting breast-feeding: The special role of maternity services.* Geneva, Switzerland: World Health Organization, p. iv.

CHAPTER 7

Assuring Ongoing Mother–Baby Contact

In hospitals and maternity care settings the world over, we've seen an impressive array of effort expended towards assuring mother–baby contact and eliminating unnecessary separation. In some settings, the struggle has been with physical space. Creative solutions have been found to relocate babies from nurseries safely within mothers' space such as "side cars" attached to mothers' bed, tables refitted with baskets, bedside baby hammocks, and lowering hospital beds by sawing off the legs.

In other settings, the issue is one of cross training or staffing. Changing care patterns may mean developing new competencies and job descriptions. Sometimes the changes revolve around acquiring a new attitude about who "owns" the baby. Institutions have to take a hard look at staffs' feeling of ownership and how this fits with the family's need to bond and learn.

As you evaluate separation of mother and baby in your setting, we suggest you use the "Process Mapping" technique described in Chapter 13. Following mothers and babies while mapping their transit through your facility can illuminate physical space, staffing, training, competency and attitude gaps, and help move the abstract concept of keeping healthy mothers and babies together to concrete strategies for change.

Optimal hospital and birth center policies and procedures promote rooming-in and eliminate routine, nonmedical occasions for separation. There should be no routine delay between the baby's birth and the initiation of continuous rooming-in. Read Box 7-1 to learn about how one hospital achieved this. Twenty-four hour rooming-in should be initiated within an hour of a vaginal birth. For mothers who give birth via cesarean, rooming-in should be started after the mother is able to respond to her baby safely. Rooming-in and on-going mother–baby contact is not just for mothers who have chosen to breastfeed their new babies. All mothers can benefit from rooming-in. Encouraging

---

Box 7-1 — The Power of Process Audit

Southside Hospital had initiated both early skin-to-skin contact and rooming-in. However a process audit indicated that there was a timing gap of an hour or more between when the mother and baby left the delivery area until they were reunited in the mother's postpartum room.

Although the transfer process for the mother was straightforward since she was rolled from the delivery area to her room, the baby had to be "admitted" through the Level 1 nursery. After transport from the delivery area to the nursery, a baby would wait until a nurse was available to go through the admission assessment and complete the paperwork. Only after this could the baby be transported to the mother's room.

The breastfeeding policy committee at Southside was surprised at the results of the process audit and discussed how to decrease the duration of the separation. The first question they explored was whether the nursery admission had to take place in the nursery. What was needed for the admission? Tools? Papers? Staff? Once it was

decided that that was not the case—the nursery was merely the traditional place that admissions had taken place—the committee decided to explore different scenarios.

The process that was ultimately decided on was to admit the baby and complete the assessment in the delivery area. Surprisingly, this change fit better into the work pattern of the nurses who would do the admission. Close to the time of birth, the nursery admissions nurse was informed of the impending event so that the admission could take place at the mother's side, usually while the baby was skin to skin. Then the mother and baby could be transported at the same time to the postpartum unit.

The Moral of the Story: Seemingly complex problems can have simple solutions when evaluated openly and critically. The first step to solving them is seeing them: it is only by examining the experience of individual mother/baby couplets that such problems become apparent.

the mother's partner to room in as well may enhance the experience.[1]

Hospital policy should provide for periodic audits of separations, and if the audit shows nonmedical occurrences, each should be investigated. Please read Box 7-2 to learn about one hospital's experience. In cases where the mother asks for a nonmedical separation, there should be documentation in the record that the mother received information about the rationale for rooming-in, and the separation should be brief, not more than 1 hour a day.

■ Why 24-Hour Rooming-In?

Mothers and Babies Can Learn Together

After the birth, mothers and babies need uninterrupted time together for skin-to-skin contact, to learn each other's cues, and to learn how to breastfeed. Twenty-four hour rooming-in is the optimal way for this learning to take place. Separation is stressful for both mother and baby, and since the time in the hospital or birth center is short, being apart from each other takes time away from essential early learning opportunities.

Being Together Fosters Closeness Between Mother and Baby

The absence of 24-hour rooming-in may have an effect on the mother's relationship with her baby. Svensson, Matthiesen, and Widström[2] concluded from their study of hospital practices that negative staff attitudes towards night rooming-in might implicitly suggest to mothers that closeness between mothers and babies is not important. Mothers who had not roomed in were more likely to believe that

---

Box 7-2	**Changing the Focus**

Achieving 24-hour rooming-in was just too hard for the staff at Bayview. The breastfeeding committee thought that rooming-in should be the first thing to accomplish after getting started at putting their breastfeeding policy into place, but the results were discouraging.

They had tried everything they could think of to deal with the barriers presented by the parents and the staff. But any gains on one month's audit of nursery use would be wiped out the next month—and then some.

The breastfeeding committee decided to change its focus to the first hour and leave achieving 24-hour rooming-in until later. They initiated skin-to-skin contact and early breastfeeding for vaginally birthing mothers first, and then for cesarean birth mothers (this was a little more complex since they recovered in a different part of the hospital).

To the committee's surprise, when they went back to audit nursery use after initiating skin-to-skin contact and early feeding, nursery use for nonmedical reasons had dropped 60%!

The Moral of the Story: Solving rooming-in barriers can be inextricably tied to both providing support during labor and assuring early contact and breastfeeding.

the staff thought their baby should stay in the nursery. Even partial (day) rooming-in had a beneficial effect in promoting a more optimal maternal–infant relationship with fewer incidences of maternal child abuse and a higher maternal attachment score at 2 to 3 days than both a pre–rooming-in group and a group who wanted rooming-in but could not have it.[3] The rate of newborn abandonment in hospital per 1000 live births was reduced from 1.8 to 0.1 two years after rooming-in was instituted in one hospital.[4]

Rooming-In Promotes Successful Breastfeeding

Rooming-in has beneficial effects both on the mother–infant relationship and on breastfeeding. Rapley,[5] commenting on the common policy of routine separation of mother and baby, asks whether it is a coincidence that breastfeeding relies on the togetherness of mother and baby! Rooming-in and the experience of rooming-in promotes successful breastfeeding,[6–15] including full or exclusive breastfeeding[16] and a longer duration of breastfeeding.[17] Perhaps this improvement in outcome is because mothers who room in produce mature milk earlier[18] and have more milk.[19] Because mothers who room in may breastfeed their babies more frequently,[20] the effect on breastfeeding outcomes may be partly because rooming-in facilitates feeding the baby on cue, at the baby's best time. When the baby spends time in the nursery, it is difficult to feed on cue. On the other hand, when babies are rooming in with their mothers, it is difficult to restrict feeds—which benefits breastfeeding outcomes.

Babies who room in with their mothers may have a lower incidence of jaundice[21] than babies who are separated from their mothers for nonmedical reasons. Even babies undergoing treatments, such as phototherapy, can room in with improved breastfeeding outcomes as measured at 4 and 12 weeks.[22]

Rooming-in babies may be also less likely to be supplemented with formula[23] and gain more weight each day in the hospital compared with separated babies.[24] However, other aspects of continuity of care, including postdischarge follow-up, are also essential in order to assure continued optimal breastfeeding practices.[25]

■ Obstacles and Solutions to Achieving 24-Hour Rooming-In

According to research into women's lived postpartum experience, the challenge to the staff is to understand the "woman as a new mother who needs both to care and be cared for both by her family and friends and by professional carers."[26]

Start With an Audit

One of the most common problems that we have noticed regarding rooming-in is that staff and administration *believe that they are practicing 24-hour rooming-in when they are not.* The only way to know whether or not babies are rooming-in with their mothers is by doing an audit of practices. The auditor should ask the question, "What percentage of babies are *not* rooming-in 24 hours a day?" Then the auditor should examine each case of separation. Was rooming-in begun shortly after delivery without a routine separation? If there was a separation, were there legitimate medical reasons for the mother and the baby to be kept apart? Was rooming-in initiated as soon as the medical indication was resolved? Or was the separation continued for arbitrary reasons (e.g., that the baby who is admitted to the nursery must stay for a minimum of 24 hours)? Is there a pattern to multiple nonmedical separations, such as nighttime separation?

Deal With the Real Concern of Staff by Examining the Evidence

Common reasons given for not rooming in, such as that it *interferes with mothers' sleep*, appear not to be valid. Another one of the concerns that is often raised about increased mother–baby contact is infection; the *fear is that rooming-in will increase the rate of nosocomial infections*. Research studies indicate that hospitals that initiate rooming-in actually have had a *reduction* in rates of infection.[27,28]

Nysaether, Baerug, Nylander, and Klepp[29] researched the common staff concern that *rooming-in might increase complaints of maternal fatigue*. They reviewed self-administered questionnaires from mothers in all Norwegian maternity wards and found no difference in tiredness between rooming-in mothers and those who chose not to have rooming-in. Another issue that usually comes up around the idea of rooming-in is the perception of staff and/or mothers that sleep quality is improved when mothers and babies are separated; mothers will get more and better rest, some think, if the baby is taken to the nursery, especially at night. The opposite is more likely (see Box 7-3).

In a research study that examined the effect of encouraging mothers to room in at

---

Box 7-3   The Safest Place for the Baby Is with the Parents

In spite of excellent security measures, Conestoga Hospital had a kidnapping near miss with a newborn baby from the Level 1 nursery. Although the baby was not removed from the hospital because a security guard stopped the perpetrator when a cry was heard from inside a bulky parka at the lobby exit, the staff was shocked. At team meetings they said to each other, "The safest place for the baby is with the parents. They shouldn't let anyone who they don't know take the baby out of their room. And even then, one parent, a grandmother, or someone should accompany the baby." This idea was repeated from one staff member to another and to every parent. "The safest place for your baby is with you, in your room. If your baby has to leave your room for a medical procedure or a check-up, we would like one of you

to always come with us. If anyone says they want you to stay here, call the desk and tell the person who answers about it."

An unintended outcome of this new staff attitude was that the nursery population decreased significantly. Only babies who needed medical care or observation while mothers received medical care were in the nursery. And beside every crib was a rocker with a family member!

The Moral of the Story: A 24-hour rooming-in goal can be accomplished as a side benefit of the desire to protect babies from kidnapping attempts. The message to parents is: "This is your baby. We want you to be part of the baby's care, in and out of your room."

night, when day rooming-in was already practiced, the findings indicated that rooming-in at night did not affect the amount of hours slept or mothers' daytime alertness, although they breastfed more frequently at night.[30]

In another study, Keefe[31] examined the nighttime sleep of a small group of mothers and the sleep-wake patterns of newborns[32] in a 24-hour rooming-in group and a group that had partial rooming-in and partial nursery use. The findings suggest that rooming-in with the baby does not greatly alter the mother's sleep, but infants' sleep is improved when they are in the room with their mothers. The researchers did not find a difference in the number of hours slept by the mothers or the quality of their sleep, although three quarters of the mothers in the partial rooming-in group took sleep medication at least once during the 2 nights of the study compared to none of the mothers in the rooming-in group. The number of infant crying episodes was greater and the caregivers responded less frequently in the nursery group.

Giving birth via a cesarean section may also be given as a reason for not instituting rooming-in care. In a study of four different pain management strategies in women who had had cesarean deliveries, pain relief was superior with a morphine regimen, and improved pain management was positively associated with breastfeeding and rooming-in.[33]

Role-playing exercises may increase staff confidence in educating mothers about rooming-in (see Box 7-4).

There may be concern about the *danger of co-sleeping*. While the 10 steps call for rooming-in, they do not require bedding-in. Many hospital beds are not safe environments for bedsharing. They are often too narrow to accommodate mother and baby comfortably and have gaps in the side rails that make them dangerous. Staff may be assured that bedding-in is not required. However, many breastfeeding mothers will end up falling asleep while holding or nursing their babies. It is crucial that mothers learn what constitutes safe co-sleep. See the resource section for more information.

Another common reason for routine separation is the perception by the staff that *routine separation is necessary for bathing, examinations, observation*, and other medical procedures. The policy development team should undertake a study of which commonly performed procedures require an infant to be taken to the nursery and which could be done in the mother's room. An advantage to doing assessments, baths, weights, and the like in the room is that there are many more occasions for education. Many facilities have put into use portable scales, bath equipment, etc. in order to be able to conduct these procedures at the mother's bedside. See Box 7-5 for one hospital's experience making these changes.

Auditing the horizontal experience of mothers and babies vis-à-vis rooming-in is a powerful action step to solving problems in this area. Because of the segmentation of hospital care, many staff are shocked to discover how much mother/baby separation goes on. Seeing the data often helps practice to change rapidly.

Resources

Academy of Breastfeeding Medicine. (n.d.). Protocol #6: Guideline on co-sleeping and breastfeeding. New Rochelle, NY: Academy of Breastfeeding Medicine. Available at http://bfmed.org/ace-files/protocol/cosleeping.pdf.

UNICEF UK Baby Friendly Initiative with the Foundation for the Study of Infant Deaths. (2005, June). Sharing a bed with your baby: A guide for mothers. London, England: UNICEF UK. Retrieved at http://

Box 7-4	**Rewriting Scripts**

The nurses at Millerstown Memorial Hospital had been working for 6 years trying to achieve 24-hour rooming-in. Month after month, year after year, the nursery was filled at night. Prenatal mother interviews consistently indicated that women who planned to deliver at Millerstown Memorial intended to room in 24 hours, yet hospital practice audits consistently indicate that fewer than 20% of mothers and babies roomed in more than 18 hours.

Jenny, the new clinical specialist, had worked previously at a hospital that had been designated a Baby-Friendly Hospital, so she knew that 24-hour rooming-in was possible. There didn't seem to be any staff resistance to the idea, they just couldn't change the practice of babies being in the nursery at night.

In a casual conversation with Marta, one of the nurses who worked overnight, Jenny brought up the subject of the babies in the nursery at night. Marta said, "I just don't know what to say to these moms when I talk to them. I ask the mother how she is. She says she's tired and needs some rest, so I say 'that's okay, I'll feed the baby in the nursery so you can get some rest.'" She continued, "I know that we want rooming-in at night. I know it's best for the babies. I know mothers sleep better and babies too. I know it's best for breastfeeding. I just don't know what to say."

This gave Jenny the idea of doing practice role plays with the nurses about what to say to a mother when she asks that her baby be taken from the postpartum room. She made up some skits (some were intentionally silly!) to get the idea across. Then there were practice sessions where the nurses worked with Jenny and with each other. The nurses reported that their confidence improved and audits showed a steady increase in the percentage of mothers rooming-in at night.

The Moral of the Story: People often know what the problem is and will tell you if you ask in a nonthreatening, nonjudgmental way. The solution to a seemingly overwhelming problem can be as simple as increasing skill and confidence through practice.

www.babyfriendly.org.uk/pdfs/sharingbedleaflet.pdf on 02/22/08.

References

1. Ringler, M., Nemeskieri, N., Uhl, A., Langer, M., & Reinold, E. (1986). Prepartale Erwartungen, Verhalten bei der Geburt und im Wochenbett sowie postpartale Zufriedenheit mit dem Geburtserlebnis [Prepartum expectations, behavior in labor and the puerperium and postpartum satisfaction with the birth experience. II. Rooming-in and breast feeding]. *Geburtshilfe und Frauenheilkunde, 46*(8), 541–544. [Article in German].
2. Svensson, K., Matthiesen, A. S., & Widstrom, A. M. (2005). Night rooming-in: Who decides? An example of staff influence on mother's attitude. *Birth, 32*(2), 99–106.
3. O'Connor, S., Vietze, P. M., Sherrod, K. B., Sandler, H. M., & Altemeier, W. A. 3rd ed. (1980). Reduced incidence of parenting inadequacy following rooming-in. *Pediatrics, 66*(2), 176–182.
4. Buranasin, B. (1991). The effects of rooming-in on the success of breastfeeding and the decline in abandonment of children. *Asia-Pacific Journal of Public Health, 5*(3), 217–220.
5. Rapley, G. (2002). Keeping mothers and babies together—breastfeeding and bonding. *Midwives Journal (Lond), 5*(10), 332–334.
6. Lin, L. C., Lee, T. Y., Kuo, S. C., Mu, P. F., & Shu, H. Q. (2004). [The lived experience of postpartum

---

Box 7-5 | Solving the Nighttime Problem

Bridgeton Hospital was working on implementing the *Ten Steps to Successful Breastfeeding* but it was stuck on 24-hour rooming-in. The problem was overnight. Although the babies stayed in the room with their mother during the daytime, when a new shift of nurses would come onto the unit in the morning, the babies were almost all in the nursery.

A survey of pregnant women who expected to deliver at Bridgeton Hospital showed that more than 80% wanted to breastfeed and not give formula at first, unless there was a medical reason, but audit reports showed that 90% sent their babies to the nursery at night. Interviews with the nurses who worked overnight indicated that mothers asked to have their babies stay in the nursery at night and be fed bottles of formula. "The mothers are tired," was the consensus statement. "They need their rest, and they are going to have to get up with the baby in the night soon enough."

After the breastfeeding committee discussed the evidence around the risks of giving babies formula for nonmedical reasons, a physician and a nurse who were members of the group volunteered to stay on the unit overnight to observe the evening and overnight breastfeeding routines.

The nighttime observers noted how many visitors the mothers had in the evening and how late they stayed. Many mothers had visitors until after 10 p.m. Then the nurses began moving the babies to the nursery for weights and other routine care. When the nurse picked up the baby she would say, "I'm taking the baby to the nursery for a weight check. What do you want me to do? Should I bring the baby back? Or do you want to sleep?" Invariably, the mothers replied that the nurse should keep the baby in the nursery because she was tired.

When the nighttime observers reported their finding back to the breastfeeding committee, a lively discussion ensued.

One person said, "I told you the mothers are tired."

Another said, "It's the visitors. We need to go back to the old way of having limited visiting hours."

Some blamed the nurses, "They should just say that the baby is coming back. Don't give the mother a choice."

After looking at the issue from all of the points of view, the committee decided to try a new procedure. The babies were weighed in the mother's room instead of the nursery in the early evening. In other words, the practice of taking the babies to the nursery late at night was dropped. The scales were easily made mobile, and the new procedure began in a week.

A month later, audits of nursery use showed that only babies whose mothers were heavily medicated for pain after cesarean births were in the nursery at night.

The Moral of the Story: Don't play the blame game. The nurses, visitors, and mothers were all blamed by someone, yet a simple change in procedure achieved the goal of 24-hour rooming-in.

women receiving rooming-in care]. *Hu Li Za Zhi,* 51(1), 35–44. [Article in Chinese].

7. McBryde, A., & Durham, N. C. (1951). Compulsory rooming-in on the ward and private newborn service at Duke Hospital. *Journal of the American Medical Association,* 145(9), 625–628.

8. Jackson, E. B., Wilkin, L. C., & Auerbach, H. (1956, May). Statistical report on incidence and duration of

breast feeding in relation to personal-social and hospital maternity factors. *Pediatrics 17*(5), 700–715.

9. Verronen, P., Visakorpi, J. K., Lammi, A., Saarikoski, S., & Taminen T. (1980). Promotion of breast feeding: Effect on neonates of change of feeding routine at a maternity unit. *Acta Paediatrica Scandinavica, 69,* 279–282.

10. Bloom, K., Goldbloom, R., Robenson, S., & Stevens, F. (1982). Factors affecting the continuance of breast feeding. *Acta Paediatrica Scandinavica, 300*(Suppl), 9–14.

11. Friedrich, W., & Beck, R. (1982). [Breast feeding under different nutritional and nursing conditions. Analysis of 644 newborn infants, 1979–1981]. *Zentralblatt für Gynäkologie, 104*(18), 1182–1192. [Article in German].

12. Gerstner, G., Kucera, H., & Kubista, E. (1983). [Breast feeding habits before and after the introduction of a partial rooming-in system]. *Geburtshilfe und Frauenheilkunde, 43*(3), 156–159. [Article in German].

13. Elander, G., & Lindberg, T. (1984). Short mother-infant separation during first week of life influences the duration of breastfeeding. *Acta Paediatrica Scandinavica, 73,* 237–240.

14. Perez-Escamilla, R., Pollitt, E., Lönnerdal, B., & Dewey, K. G. (1994). Infant feeding policies in maternity wards and their effect on breast-feeding success: An analytical overview. *American Journal of Public Health, 84*(1), 89–97.

15. Procianoy, R. S., Fernandes-Filho, P. H., Lazaro, L., Sartori, N.C., & Drebes, S. (1983). The influence of rooming-in on breastfeeding. *Journal of Tropical Pediatrics, 29,* 112–114.

16. Strachan-Lindenberg, C., Cabrera-Artola, R., & Jimenez, V. (1990). The effect of early post-partum mother-infant contact and breastfeeding promotion on the incidence and continuation of breast-feeding. *International Journal of Nursing Studies, 27*(3), 179–186.

17. Daglas, M., Antoniou, E., Pitselis, G., Iatrakis, G., Kourounis, G., & Ccreatsas, G. (2005). Factors influencing the initiation and progress of breastfeeding in Greece. *Clinical and Experimental Obstetrics & Gynecology, 32*(3), 189–192.

18. Mapata, S., Djauhariah, A. M., & Dasril, D. (1988). A study comparing rooming-in with separate nursing. *Paediatrica Indonesiana, 28,* 116–123.

19. Aisaka, K., Mori, H., Ogawa, T., & Kigawa, T. (1985). [Effects of mother-infant interaction on maternal milk secretion and dynamics of maternal serum prolactin levels in puerperium]. *Nippon Sanka Fujinka Gakkai Zasshi, 37*(5), 713–720. [Article in Japanese].

20. Perez-Escamilla, R., Segura-Millán, S., Pollitt, E., & Dewey, K.G. (1992). Effect of the maternity ward system on the lactation success of low-income urban Mexican women. *Early Human Development, 31,* 25–40.

21. Mapata, S., Djauhariah, A. M., & Dasril, D. (1988). A study comparing rooming-in with separate nursing. *Paediatrica Indonesiana, 28,* 116–123.

22. Elander, G., & Lindberg, T. (1986). Hospital routines in infants with hyperbilirubinemia influence the duration of breastfeeding. *Acta Paediatrica Scandinavica, 75,* 708–712.

23. Pechlivani, F., Vassilakou, T., Sarafidou, J., Zachou, T., Anastasiou, C. A., & Sidossis, L. S. (2005). Prevalence and determinants of exclusive breast-feeding during hospital stay in the area of Athens, Greece. *Acta Paediatrica, 94*(7), 928–934.

24. Yamauchi, Y., & Yamanouchi, I. (1990) The relationship between rooming-in/not rooming-in and breast-feeding variables. *Acta Paediatrica Scandinavica, 79,* 1017–1022.

25. Perez-Escamilla, R., Segura-Millán, S., Pollitt, E., & Dewey, K.G. (1992). Effect of the maternity ward system on the lactation success of low-income urban Mexican women. *Early Human Development, 31,* 25–40.

26. Bondas-Salonen, T. (1998, March). New mothers' experiences of postpartum care—a phenomenological follow-up study. *Journal of Clinical Nursing, 7*(2), 165.

27. Mapata, S., Djauhariah, A. M., & Dasril, D. (1988). A study comparing rooming-in with separate nursing. *Paediatrica Indonesiana, 28,* 116–123.

28. Suradi, R. (1988), Rooming-in for babies born by caesarean section in Dr. Cipto Mangunkusumo General Hospital Jakarta. *Paediatrica Indonesiana, 28,* 124–132.

29. Nysaether, H., Baerug, A., Nylander, G., & Klepp, K. I. (2002). *Barna inne natt og dag—er barselkvinnene fornøyde?* [Rooming-in in the maternity ward—are mothers satisfied?]. *Tidsskrift for den Norske laegeforening, 112*(12), 1206–1209. [Article in Norwegian].

30. Waldenstrom, U., & Swenson, A. (1991). Rooming-in at night in the postpartum ward. *Midwifery, 7,* 82–89.

31. Keefe, M. R. (1988, March–April). The impact of infant rooming-in on maternal sleep at night. *Journal of Obstetrics, Gynecology and Neonatal Nursing, 17*(2), 122–126.

32. Keefe, M. R. (1987). Comparison of neonatal nighttime sleep-wake patterns in nursery versus rooming-in environments. *Nursing Research, 36*(3), 140–144.

33. Yost, N. P., Bloom, S. L., Sibley, M. K., Lo, J. Y., McIntire, D. D., & Leveno, K. J. (2004). A hospital-sponsored quality improvement study of pain management after cesarean delivery. *American Journal of Obstetrics & Gynecology, 190*(5), 1341–1346.

CHAPTER

8

Pacing the Breastfeedings

■ The Argument for Breastfeeding on Demand

Achieving continuity of care around breast-feeding management requires agreement on the part of staff members that breastfeeding is normal, desirable, and achievable. Feeding babies at predetermined and regular intervals must be confronted as an artifact of formula feeding and replaced with an agreement that irregular, clustered, and frequent feeding at the breast is optimal. Letting go of formulas' "clock-watching" and substituting "baby-watching" requires knowledge, practice, and attitude changes on the part of the staff.

Breastfeeding on demand (when the baby shows feeding cues) has clear benefits compared to scheduled feedings and has been described and recommended as the optimal breastfeeding strategy for many years.[1–6] Studies of breastfeeding on demand also show that there is increased weight gain in the newborn[7,8] compared with the weight gain of babies fed according to a set schedule, as well as a longer duration of breastfeeding,[9,10] and a greater probability of breastfeeding exclusively.[11,12]

Mothers usually need encouragement to *watch the baby, not the clock,* in order to know when it's time to feed the baby and when the feeding should end. Breastfeeding works best when the mother and her supporters understand that newborn babies are expected to breastfeed a minimum of 10 to 12 times in 24 hours. The range of 30–36 breastfeedings in the first 3 days is associated with a decrease in hyperbilirubinemia compared to infants with fewer (24–29) feedings.[13] Other studies have confirmed that implementing frequent breastfeedings is related to decreased risk of hyperbilirubunemia.[14,15]

During the hospital stay, unrestricted feeding is really only feasible in concert with achieving a goal of 24-hour rooming-in, which enables the mother to respond when her infant shows readiness to feed. Feeding on demand should be the standard of practice for all families, whether breastfeeding or formula-feeding. When the breastfeeding mother and baby respond to each other they can achieve nutritional homeostasis, according to researchers who found that the interval between feedings decreased between day 1 and day 2 and that weight gain occurred at day 3. They also report that the baby exhibited an increased drive to eat when weight loss exceeds 6%. After a 10% weight loss, there was a further 7% shortening of the interval between feedings.[16] The researchers concluded that breastfeeding on demand is accompanied by a balanced nutritional status.

■ Is There a Downside to Encouraging Unrestricted Breastfeeding?

In the past, there were concerns that unrestricted breastfeeding could have untoward effects, such as an increased risk of sore nipples, but research indicates that sore nipples are mainly due to poor attachment at the breast.[17–19] A systematic review of research related to newborn feeding schedules in the hospital setting concluded that restricted breastfeeding was associated with an increased incidence of sore nipples, an increased incidence of engorgement, and an increased need to give additional formula feeds.[20]

■ Feeding on Cue

Breastfeeding on demand works best when mothers are encouraged to feed their babies in

---

Box 8-1	**Early Feeding Cues**

- Rooting, turning the head especially with searching movements of the mouth
- Increasing alertness, especially rapid eye movement under closed eyelids
- Flexing of the legs and arms
- Bringing or attempting to bring a hand to the mouth (the baby does not have to be successful)
- Sucking on a fist or finger
- Mouthing motions of the lips and tongue
- Head bobbing

response to the baby's signs of feeding readiness, or feeding cues. But first, the mother and her supporters need teaching in order to learn how to recognize early feeding cues and help to understand that crying is a late feeding cue (see Box 8-1). There is no regular time interval expected between feedings, so mothers should not be given instruction to nurse every 2, 2½, or 3 hours or at any time interval.

The Baby Ends the Feeding

Feedings also vary in length, with the baby expected to end the feeding by releasing the nipple, relaxing the body, and (sometimes) making small, satisfied sounds. Mothers should *not* be instructed to nurse the baby 10, 15, 20, or any number of minutes on each side. Babies should nurse until they are finished on one breast. Then the mother should offer the other breast. Some babies will want to nurse right away on the second side while others rest or sleep between breasts. Questions have also arisen about whether staff should encourage mothers to feed from one or both breasts at each feeding, but experimental designed studies[21,22] indicate that the baby's appetite should be the deciding factor. As the early days pass and the milk changes from colostrum to mature milk, the mother and her baby will develop the pattern that is right for them.

The feeding should end when the baby latches off on his or her own. The baby's hands will be open and the arms will be limp. The body tone will be soft. If one hand is limp and the other clenched and tight when the baby latches off, the baby will usually want to nurse again in a little while.

Irregular Time Intervals Are to Be Expected

Breastfeedings are usually not spaced evenly around the clock. Babies, especially newly born babies, typically cluster feed. That is, they have several nursings close together and then space other nursings further apart. At first, days and nights are mixed up for many babies, but if the mother pays attention to feeding cues in the daytime and nurses frequently according to the baby's cues, the nighttime feedings will begin to space out.

How Long Does a Breastfeeding Last?

As a general rule, full-term newborns can efficiently and effectively transfer milk faster than babies born close to term (near-term). As a group, prematurely born babies transfer milk at the slowest rate.

After the early days, full-term efficient and effective nursers take between 15 and 20 minutes to feed. If a baby is full term, more than 4 days old, and nurses more than 20 minutes or less than 15, that is one sign that an individualized breastfeeding assessment from a breastfeeding caregiver or healthcare provider is needed. Before-and-after weights using a digital scale accurate to 2 grams will allow the breastfeeding care-giver or health-care provider to estimate the amount of milk transferred.

Contrary to popular belief, babies who nurse for longer times often transfer less milk than babies who nurse around 15 to 20 minutes. Research indicates that babies who are not effective and efficient in milk transfer actually give their mother's breasts and hormones the message to make *less* milk over time.[23]

■ Will the Baby Get Enough Fat?

Babies need the fat in breast milk for their body functions, brain, and nervous system development and energy. Today, because of excellent research studies, we have a better understanding of fat and breastfeeding.

The Old Idea

In the past, people had the idea that the milk at the end of the nursing, the hind milk, was always higher in fat than the rest of the milk, and always higher in fat than the milk at the beginning of the feeding, the fore milk. So, people thought that each breastfeeding should last a long time so that the baby would get to the hind milk. If a baby was not gaining enough weight, mothers were told to make the nursing last longer.

The New Idea

Our new understanding, based on well-done research,[24] indicates that babies get ideal amounts of fat with effective and efficient breastfeedings, not according to how long the nursing lasts or how many feedings there are.

We now know that sometimes the milk at the end of a nursing is higher in fat and sometimes it's not. Sometimes the fat in the milk at the beginning and the end of the breastfeeding is about the same. We know that the proportion of fat and the volume of milk vary by the time of day (more fat in the evening, higher volume in the morning). We know that fat is related more to the volume of milk than to how long the feeding lasts.

Another finding is that the speed of milk removal influences the amount of fat in the milk; so effective, efficient breastfeedings are best. When the speed and efficiency of the feeding are improved, there will be increased fat in the milk. Of course, it takes time for newborn babies to learn to feed efficiently. For this reason, it is crucial that trained staff assess multiple feedings to assure the growing skill of the mother and baby.

■ Pacing the Feedings From Self-Attached to Collaborative Breastfeeding[25]

Normal breastfeeding progresses through two phases. In the first phase, the baby latches to the breast without assistance and self-attaches to the breast using the stepping-crawling reflex; this is *self-attached breastfeeding*. In the second phase, the mother and baby work together to achieve the latch and feeding: *collaborative breastfeeding*.

Hospital and birth center policies should encourage *skin-to-skin* holding soon after birth (see Chapter 4) and move to *self-attached breastfeeding* where the baby takes the lead. This often happens within the first hour or 2 after birth. Research indicates that when babies have had the opportunity to move to the breast and begin nursing by self-attaching, they have a better latch.[26] *Self-attached breastfeeding* uses the baby's innate skill and ability to locate the nipple and begin breastfeeding. *Collaborative breastfeeding* is more of what people imagine breastfeeding to be—the mother and baby work to achieve breastfeeding together. In the first days, mothers should gradually increase the number of *collaborative breastfeedings* where she and the baby work together.

Self-Attached Breastfeeding

Self-attached breastfeeding should begin as soon as possible after birth and can continue as the primary mode of latching on during the first days, gradually giving way to a collaborative feeding mode.

Self-attached feeding begins with skin-to-skin holding and allows the baby to use a stepping-crawling motion to approach the breast, nuzzle, and nurse. This journey may take more than 2 hours if the mother has received drugs in labor, less if she has not. If the birth was by cesarean section, skin-to-skin holding and self-attached breastfeeding can begin as soon as the mother is ready, in the delivery room, in the recovery area, or in her hospital room. Until the mother is ready, the father or another adult can hold the baby skin to skin.

To begin skin-to-skin holding, the healthy baby is dried off and put on the mother's chest. The baby is usually positioned between the mother's breasts. Both mother and baby are then covered with a warmed blanket and a cap is placed on the baby's head. The baby goes through stages of awakening and approaches the breast using a stepping-crawling motion, massaging the fundus with the knees and feet. The baby will locate the breast, nuzzle, and ideally, find the nipple and self-attach.

The baby is preferentially attracted to the odor of human milk over the odor of formula,[27] including the odor from the skin glands of the mother's areolae.[28] Exposure to the mother's odor may also facilitate the infant's adaptation to the early postnatal en-

vironment.[29] The mother's areolae and milk odor appear to be enough of an incentive to attract and guide the newly born baby to the breast[30] especially after the infant has been exposed to the contractions of labor.[31] Mother–infant skin-to-skin contact for more than 50 minutes immediately after birth may result in enhanced infant recognition of his or her own mother's milk odor and result in a longer duration of breastfeeding.[32] Skin-to-skin contact is also an opportunity for the mother's body to warm the baby. She actually does this better than hospital warming cots or cribs, according to research.[33] The mother's breasts will increase and decrease temperature[34] according to the infant's needs.

Sometimes mothers and staff get the impression that skin-to-skin contact is a procedure only for the first hours of life. On the contrary, skin-to-skin contact should continue as a method of calming and connecting with baby for as long as mother and baby wish.

Collaborative Breastfeeding

With collaborative breastfeeding, as the baby seeks the breast, the mother gently assists. The mother uses her body, arms, hands, and lap to hold the baby. The mother should initiate collaborative breastfeeding when she feels ready and continue self-attached feedings to assure adequate intake for the infant. A suggestion for postures and instructions for mothers may be found in Boxes 8-2 and 8-3.

■ Overcoming Common Barriers to Implementation

Frequent breastfeeding, on demand, is associated with lowering the risk of jaundice in

Box 8-2   Feeding Observation Checklist

Before the feed:

☐ If available, weigh baby prior to feeding on a digital scale, sensitive to 2 grams. Baby need not be naked, but should be weighed after the feeding in the same clothes, without diaper changing.

☐ Does skin-to-skin contact precede the feeding?

☐ What cues does mother respond to in deciding when to feed?

☐ Is the baby too hungry to feed well (e.g., frantic, crying)?

☐ Is the baby not hungry at all (e.g., deeply sleeping, shutdown)?

☐ How does mother prepare for the feed?

☐ How much time lapses from observed cues until baby is brought to the breast?

☐ Position yourself so that you can best view the feeding from the mother's perspective. For example, standing behind the mother as shown in **Figure B-1**.

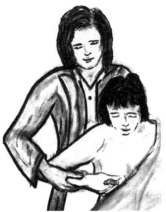

Figure B-1 When the helper stands behind the mother and looks over her shoulder, she sees the mother's view of what is happening. *Source*: Healthy Children Project

As the baby latches:

☐ What does the nipple look like before it enters the baby's mouth? Note shape and coloration.

☐ What position does the mother choose?

☐ Is baby's body turned toward mother?

☐ Is baby's body aligned (ears over shoulders, shoulders over hips, legs and arms flexed to midline)?

☐ Where are mother's hands?

☐ Does she have her hand on the back of the baby's head or the sides of the baby's face?

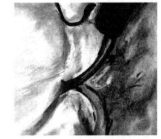

Figure B-2 Poor Latch: Baby's mouth is latched to the breast at a 90-degree angle. *Source*: Healthy Children Project

☐ Is she using her hand to alter the natural shape of the breast and/or the tilt of the nipple? What is baby's position relative to the mother's nipple?

☐ When does baby open mouth?

☐ What is angle of mouth opening? For example, the baby in **Figure B-2** has a mouth opening angle of approximately 90 degrees, too small for effective, comfortable feeding.

☐ Does mother respond to wide-open mouth by drawing baby in close?

☐ Is baby able to extend the head backward? Or is the head being held toward the baby's chest?

☐ Does baby reach breast with lower lip and tongue first, followed by the upper lip sealing to the breast?

☐ Does baby's mouth appear off-center in relation to the position of the nipple?

☐ Is baby's chin dug into the breast?

☐ Is baby's nose near the breast?

/continues

Box 8-2　**Feeding Observation Checklist (continued)**

During the feed:

☐ Observe mother's body language while feeding. Look for tension in arms, shoulders, hands, feet, and face.

☐ Observe baby's body language while feeding. Look for signs of tension or distress.

☐ Is the motion of the baby's jaw an up-and-down piston motion as in **Figure B-3**? If so, this is correlated with nonnutritive sucking.

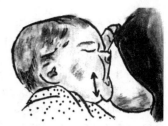

Figure B-3 Piston motion of the jaw is associated with nonnutritive sucking. *Source*: Healthy Children Project

☐ Is the motion of the baby's jaw moving in a rocker-like fashion as in **Figure B-4**, with the jaw driving forward into the breast? If so, this is correlated with nutritive sucking.

☐ How does baby handle the milk flow?

☐ Does baby sputter or choke during the feeding?

☐ Does baby stay at the breast or come off and on during the feed?

☐ Does baby seem to have difficulty breathing at the breast?

☐ Does the skin around the baby's mouth and nose appear normal during the feeding? (Blue coloration is a sign of a medical problem—ensure immediate comprehensive pediatric exam).

☐ Count rhythm of sucks to swallows.

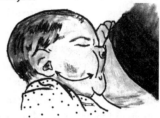

Figure B-4 Rocker motion of the jaw is associated with nutritive sucking. *Source*: Healthy Children Project

After the feed:

☐ What triggers the end of the feed (the clock, the mother's determination the feed is over, the baby's self removal)?

☐ What does the mother's nipple look like just as it exits the baby's mouth? Any change in shape (other than increased length and width)?

☐ Any change in coloration of the nipple?

the baby as well as promoting optimal breastfeeding outcomes. Although hospital or birth center policy may state that babies are to be fed according to the baby's cue, and that babies should be fed 10–12 times a day, there may be a gap between policy and practice.

An *audit process* should be instituted in order to determine whether on-demand, cue-based breastfeedings are the instituted norm and whether or not the staff are skilled in supporting the practice. An audit that interviews mothers will reveal what they and their supporters have learned during their postpartum stay. Demand feeding may be specified but written materials or staff[35] may suggest teaching the newborn a schedule before he or she leaves the hospital (see Box 8-4).

Unfortunately, decades of formula use and scheduled feeding policies have led to the expectation on the part of mothers and

Box 8-3   **Instructions for Mothers for Collaborative Feedings**

- Observe for feeding cues. Try to begin with an early cue, such as rapid eye movement.
- Wash your hands.
- Get comfortable in the posture of your choice and put the baby close to your breast in the position of your choice. Free your breast. Be sure your bra is not pressing anywhere on your breast.
- There is usually no need to hold your breast during the nursing. If you wish to support your breast, it's best to do so in a way that keeps your fingers away from the nipple and also does not put pressure on the ducts. A good way to do this is to put your hand flat against your chest, under your breast, with your thumb up and over your breast. Make your hand come up as high as possible into the crease. This will bring your breast out away from your chest. Another way to accomplish the same thing is to roll a facecloth or small towel and put it under your breast as high as possible.
- Use your hand to cup the baby's shoulders and the base of the baby's neck (not the back of the head).
- The baby's arm shouldn't be crossed in front of the body or swaddled. Let the arms be out and up around the breast, almost like a hug.
- The baby should be tummy to tummy with you.
- Start with the baby's nose opposite your nipple.
- Bring the baby back away from the breast (about 1–3 inches).
- As the baby mouth opens wide (gapes), the head will tilt back slightly during the latch. Be sure there is no pressure against the back of the baby's head.
- Move the baby to the breast. Do not direct the breast to the baby. In the football or the cross-cradle hold, your hand on the base of

the neck is bringing the baby in to you. If you are holding the baby in a cradle hold, hold the baby's head on your forearm, not in the crook of your elbow, and bring your arm in to bring the baby to breast. The nipple has to be positioned between the tongue and the roof of the mouth, so bringing the baby to the nipple works best.

- The tongue extends over the lower lip and the chin reaches the breast first. The baby's mouth is wide open as it reaches the breast.
- The latch should be asymmetrical. More of the top of the areola may be showing and less of the bottom of the areola will be visible.
- The lips should make a seal around the breast. They may look flanged, sort of like a fish, but not so flanged that the gums, rather than the lips are making contact with the breast. The tongue should be stretched forward over the lower gum line.
- The nose should be close to the breast. The chin may be closer, touching or digging into the breast, due to the head tilt.
- The corner of the baby's mouth will make an angle greater than 140°.
- The cheeks will look full, not dimpled or drawn in.
- The baby begins to suck and swallow. The jaw motion should extend back to the baby's ear. After the first few days, you will hear the baby swallow.
- Breastfeeding should not hurt if the baby is latched correctly. At the most, you might feel a gentle tugging. At the end of the feeding your nipple should be shaped as it was before baby latched on.

In addition, assessment of the feeding by a skilled observer should indicate that the nursing has efficiently and effectively transferred milk.

staff that feeding should occur on a regular, predictable schedule. *Staff training and ori-* *entations* should include a discussion of the advantages of the institution's unrestricted

---

| **Box 8-4** | **Watch Out for Mixed Messages** |

Sylvan Hospital, located in an affluent suburban community with well-insured, highly educated clients, had a breastfeeding initiation rate of over 80%. Sylvan's breastfeeding committee and staff had worked for 3 years to improve the breastfeeding environment and patient outcomes as the hospital worked toward becoming designated as a Baby-Friendly hospital. After submitting its self-assessment and fulfilling the other required procedures, Sylvan received a certificate of intent from Baby-Friendly USA, the agency responsible to WHO and UNICEF for implementing the Baby-Friendly Hospital Initiative in the United States. The hospital staff then began to assure themselves that all 10 steps to successful breastfeeding were in place.

Sylvan's to-do list included instituting rooming-in, early skin-to-skin holding, self-attachment, and decreasing the use of nonmedical formula supplementation with breastfed babies. All of the nurses and ancillary staff received breastfeeding training that encouraged, among the other topics suggested by WHO/UNICEF and Baby-Friendly USA, feeding on cue without restrictions. When the nurses were audited, it was clear that their practices supported the hospital's breastfeeding policy.

Sylvan's quality improvement department was charged with the job of monitoring two outcomes, the amount of supplementary formula given to breastfed babies and the jaundice diagnosis rate of babies before and after the policy and training portion of the new policy was implemented. The breastfeeding committee had looked forward, learning from the quality improvement study that the rate of supplementation and the number of babies with jaundice had decreased. Unfortunately, the supplementation rate only went down a small amount and the jaundice rate hadn't gone down at all.

Baby-Friendly USA encouraged the breastfeeding committee to audit practice further by interviewing pregnant women and mothers in the hospital, both on the first and second day after giving birth, about their breastfeeding intentions. The pregnant women who were interviewed reported that babies should be breastfed on demand, although they couldn't name any feeding cues or indicators of demand except crying. By the second day in the hospital, the postpartum mothers told the audit team that babies should be breastfed every 3 hours for 10 minutes on each breast. The team realized that in spite of the breastfeeding policy and trainings, the message of scheduled feedings was strongly disseminated to the mothers after admission.

Where were these messages coming from? One mother explained to the interviewer, "The nurses explained about feeding cues and all, but the handout about breastfeeding and the TV show on the hospital station said that it was best to put the baby on a schedule, every 2½ to 3 hours and not to let the baby nurse more than 10 minutes on each side otherwise you would get sore nipples."

The Moral of the Story: Television and written materials can be a powerful influence and must be examined for their congruency with healthcare provider teaching.

feeding policy and also provide practical, how-to information that assures that staff can recognize and teach feeding cues[36] and assess a breastfeeding, including assuring optimal latch. Staff should also be prepared to support self-attached breastfeedings that begin right after the birth and continue during the postpartum stay as the mother and baby learn to collaboratively feed.

■ Assure 24-Hour Rooming-In

Unrestricted breastfeeding requires unrestricted access. When the mother and baby are separated by rules, by interruptions, by visitors, by distance, or by misconception, frequent unrestricted breastfeeding is not possible. Quality improvement projects, practice audits, and patient outcomes should be routinely monitored in order to assure frequent, unrestricted breastfeeding.

Resources

The low-cost patient education materials below were developed by the Healthy Children Project's Center for Breastfeeding and are available from Health Education Associates:

How to Hold Your Baby Skin-to-Skin (a tear-off pad which explains the benefits of holding the baby skin-to-skin in the hospital for term babies, in the special care nursery and at home)

Breastfeeding Latch-On 1,2,3 (a full color tear-off pad with photographs to help mothers latch their baby on to their breast) Available in several languages.

Feeding Cues for Breastfed Babies and Mother's Breastfeeding Log (a tear-off pad which helps mothers learn about feeding cues on one side, with a breastfeeding log for the first week after birth on the other side) Available in English and Spanish.

Lactation Assessment and Comprehensive Intervention Tool (The LAT) (A comprehensive NCR—one for the record, one for the mother—form that includes the ideal assessment findings as well as check-off boxes for observed behavior. Elements include feeding cues, latching process, angle of mouth opening, flanging of lips, positioning, and rhythm.)

References

1. Cruse, P., Yudkin, P., & Baum, J. D. (1978). Establishing demand feeding in hospital. *Archives of Diseases in Childhood, 53*(1), 76–78.
2. Fisher, C. (1985). The puerperium and breastfeeding. In G. N. Marsh (Ed.), *Modern Obstetrics in General Practice*. Oxford, England: Oxford University Press. p. 325–348.
3. Klaus, M. H. (1987). The frequency of suckling. *Obstetrics and Gynecology Clinics of North America, 14*(3), 623–633.
4. Inch, S., & Garforth, S. (1989). Establishing and maintaining breastfeeding. In I. Chalmers, M. W. Enkin, & M. Kierse (Eds.), *Effective Care in Pregnancy and Childbirth*. Oxford, England: Oxford University Press. p. 1359–1374.
5. Slaven, S., & Harvey, D. (1981). Unlimited suckling time improves breast feeding. *Lancet, I*(8216), 392–393.
6. de Carvalho, M., Robertson, S., & Klaus, M. H. (1984). Does the duration and frequency of early breastfeeding affect nipple pain? *Birth, 11*, 81–84.
7. de Carvalho, M., Robertson, S., Friedman, A., & Klaus, M. (1983). Effect of frequent breast-feeding on early milk production and infant weight gain. *Pediatrics, 72*(3), 307–311.
8. Illingworth, R. S., & Stone, D. G. H. (1952). Self-demand feeding in a maternity unit. *Lancet, I*(6710), 683–687.
9. Labarere, J., Dalla-Lana, C., Schelstraete, C., Rivier, A., Callec, M., Polverelli, J. F., et al. (2001). Initiation et durée de l'allaitement maternel dans les établissements d'Aix et Chambéry (France) [Initiation and duration of breastfeeding in obstetrical hospitals in Aix-Chambery (France)]. *Archives de Pédiatrie, 8*(8), 807–815. [Article in French].
10. Martines, J. C., Ashworth, A., & Kirkwood, B. (1989). Breast-feeding among the urban poor in southern Brazil: Reasons for termination in the first 6 months of life. *Bulletin of the World Health Organization, 67*(2), 151–161.
11. Kurinij, N., & Shiono, P. H. (1991). Early formula supplementation of breast-feeding. *Pediatrics, 88*(4), 745–750.
12. Pechlivani, F., Vassilakou, T., Sarafidou, J., Zachou, T., Anastasiou, C. A., Sidossis, L. S., et al. (2005).

Prevalence and determinants of exclusive breast-feeding during hospital stay in the area of Athens, Greece. *Acta Paediatrica, 94*(7), 928–934.

13. Varimo, P., Simila, S., Wendt, L., & Kolvisto, M. (1986, February). Frequency of breast-feeding and hyperbilirubinemia. *Clinical Pediatrics (Phila.), 25*(2), 112.

14. de Carvalho, M., Klaus, M. H., & Merkatz, R. B. (1982). Frequency of breast-feeding and serum bilirubin concentration. *American Journal of Diseases of Children, 136*, 737–738.

15. Yamauchi, Y., & Yamanouchi, I. (1990). Breast-feeding frequency during the first 24 hours after birth in full-term neonates. *Pediatrics, 86*(2), 171–175.

16. Marchini, G., Persson, B., Berggren, V., & Hagenäs, L. (1998). Hunger behaviour contributes to early nutritional homeostasis. *Acta Paediatrica, 87*(6), 671–675.

17. Cadwell, K., Turner-Maffei, C., Blair, A., Brimdyr, K., & McInerney, Z. M. (2004). Pain reduction and treatment of sore nipples in nursing mothers. *Journal of Perinatal Education, 13*(1), 29–34.

18. Blair, A., Cadwell, K., Turner-Maffei, C., Brimdyr, K., & McInenerny, Z. (2003). The relationship between positioning, the breastfeeding dynamic, the latching process and pain in breastfeeding mothers with sore nipples. *Breastfeeding Review, 11*(2), 5–10.

19. Salomon, C. W., Wegnelius, G., Holmgren-Lie, A., Kolskog, E., & Jonsson, G. (2000). Seven years experience at a specialized breastfeeding clinic. Incorrect breastfeeding technique and milk stasis are the most common problems. *Lakartidningen, 97*(43), 4838–4842.

20. Renfrew, M. J., Lang, S., Martin, L., & Woolridge, M. W. (2000). Feeding schedules in hospitals for newborn infants. *Cochrane Database of Systematic Reviews,* (2), CD000090.

21. Evans, K., Evans, R., & Simmer, K. (1995). Effect of the method of breast feeding on breast engorgement, mastitis and infantile colic. *Acta Paediatrica, 84*(8), 849–852.

22. Righard, L., Flodmark, C. E., Lothe, L., & Jakobsson, I. (1993). Breastfeeding patterns: Comparing the effects on infant behavior and maternal satisfaction of using one or two breasts. *Birth, 20*(4), 182–185.

23. Kent, J. C. (2007, November–December). How breastfeeding works. *Journal of Midwifery and Women's Health, 52*(6), 564–570.

24. Kent, J. C., Mitoulas, L. R., Cregan, M. D., Ramsay, D. T., Doherty, D. A., & Hartmann, P. E. (2006, March). Volume and frequency of breastfeedings and fat content of breast milk throughout the day. *Pediatrics, 117*(3), e387–e395.

25. Cadwell, K.(2007). Latching-on and suckling of the healthy term neonate: Breastfeeding assessment. *Journal of Midwifery and Women's Health, 52*(6), 638–642.

26. Righard, L., & Alade, M. O. (1990). Effect of delivery room routines on success of first breast-feed. *Lancet, 336*(8723), 1105–1107.

27. Marlier, L., & Schaal, B. (2005, January–February). Human newborns prefer human milk: Conspecific milk odor is attractive without postnatal exposure. *Child Development, 76*(1), 155–168.

28. Schaal, B., Doucet, S., Sagot, P., Hertling, E., & Soussignan, R. (2006, March). Human breast areolae as scent organs: Morphological data and possible involvement in maternal-neonatal co-adaptation. *Devopmental Psychobiology, 48*(2), 100–110.

29. Porter, R. H. (2004, December). The biological significance of skin-to-skin contact and maternal odours. *Acta Paediatrica, 93*(12), 1560–1562.

30. Varendi, H., & Porter, R. H. (2001, April). Breast odour as the only maternal stimulus elicits crawling towards the odour source. *Acta Paediatrica, 90*(4), 372–375.

31. Varendi, H., Porter, R. H., & Winberg, J. (2002, April). The effect of labor on olfactory exposure learning within the first postnatal hour. *Behavioral Neuroscience, 116*(2), 206–211.

32. Mizuno, K., Mizuno, N., Shinohara, T., & Noda, M. (2004, December). Mother-infant skin-to-skin contact after delivery results in early recognition of own mother's milk odour. *Acta Paediatrica, 93*(12), 1640–1645.

33. Christensson, K., Siles, C., Moreno, L., Belaustequi, A., De La Fuente, P., Lagercrantz, H., et al. (1992, Jun–Jul). Temperature, metabolic adaptation and crying in healthy full-term newborns cared for skin-to-skin or in a cot. *Acta Paediatrica, 81*(6–7), 488–493.

34. Kimura, C., & Matsuoka, M. (2007, February). Changes in breast skin temperature during the course of breastfeeding. *Journal of Human Lactation, 23*(1), 60–69.

35. Garforth, S., & Garcia, J. (1989). Breast feeding policies in practice—"No wonder they get confused." *Midwifery, 5*, 75–83.

36. Marasco, L., & Barger, J. (1999). Cue feeding: Wisdom and science. *Breastfeeding Abstracts, 18*(4), 28–29.

Ten Steps to Successful Breastfeeding
A Joint WHO/UNICEF Statement[a]

Every facility providing maternity services and care for newborn infants should:

1. Have a written breastfeeding policy that is routinely communicated to all healthcare staff.
2. Train all healthcare staff in skills necessary to implement this policy.
3. Inform all pregnant women about the benefits and management of breastfeeding.
4. Help mothers initiate breastfeeding within a half-hour of birth. (US, one hour)
5. Show mothers how to breastfeed, and how to maintain lactation even if they should be separated from their infants.
6. Give newborn infants no food or drink other than breastmilk unless medically indicated.
7. Practice rooming in—allow mothers and infants to remain together—24 hours a day.
8. Encourage breastfeeding on demand.
9. **Give no artificial teats (US, nipples) or pacifiers (also called dummies or soothers) to breastfeeding infants.**
10. Foster the establishment of breastfeeding support groups and refer mothers to them on discharge from the hospital or clinic.

---

[a] World Health Organization. (1989). *Protecting, promoting and supporting breast-feeding: The special role of maternity services.* Geneva, Switzerland: World Health Organization, p. iv.

CHAPTER 9

Avoiding Extracurricular Suckling and Feeding in the Learning Phase of Breastfeeding

It's not unusual for maternity care facilities to uncover conflict around the use of pacifiers (also called "dummies") and bottles and bottle nipples (sometimes referred to as "teats.") Some staff members may have used pacifiers and baby bottles for their own children and may feel defensive about their own parenting decisions when policy and practice restrict their use. We have heard "I breastfed and used a pacifier (or bottle) with my baby and everything turned out fine" more times than can be counted. As you work to achieve continuity of care around breastfeeding, you will hear it too!

We've found that responding in a personal way, but delineating between personal experience and professional practice, can be both caring and effective. "I'm glad that it worked out for you and your family, but when we are making policy and thinking about our practice, we have to think of the larger population and what will work best in terms of a public health strategy. Please support our new policy."

In the early days of breastfeeding, the baby and mother are learning the intimate dance of feeding. During this time, it is best to avoid introduction of pacifiers or bottle-feeding to the breastfed baby, as such other suckling and feeding experiences expose the baby to different shapes of teats, different types of fluids, and different transfer actions.

In the past, it was said that newborn breastfed babies who had suckled on artificial teats (the international term for pacifiers and bottle nipples) were at risk of developing nipple confusion. Neifert, Lawrence, and Seacat sought to develop a formal definition of this condition.[1] Other infant feeding experts have questioned this terminology, wondering if nipple confusion truly exists or is rather an excuse given by those with inadequate skill at assisting a distressed baby in achieving comfort at the breast.[2] Some babies do appear less able or willing to sense the softer more pliable shape of their mother's nipple in their mouth after feeling the harder, firmer shape of the artificial teat. Woolridge has referred to the larger, firmer shape of the artificial teat as a supernormal stimulus to the baby.[3]

Clearly, many babies appear to have no difficulty going between the bottle and the breast. However, it is not possible to predict exactly which babies will have such difficulty. Thus, it is optimal to avoid pacifiers and bottles during the early weeks of breastfeeding.

The major differences between suckling on the breast and suckling on the bottle appear to be the degree of expansion of the teat[b] inside the baby's mouth[4,5] and the sucking pattern and amount of negative pressure generated in the baby's mouth.[6]

Negative pressure, or suction, helps the milk to flow from both the breast and the bottle. Very little milk flows on compression of either breast or the bottle nipple.[7] The first stage of suckling involves creating a seal by attaching the lips firmly to the surface of the breast or bottle. The tongue and jaw drop, creating a vacuum (negative pressure). The teat expands into this space and the vacuum encourages milk to flow. The baby lowers and raises the jaw, increasing and decreasing the negative pressure. A bolus of milk forms at the back of the tongue, triggering swallowing when it reaches critical mass.

In breastfeeding, the mother's milk ejection reflex works with the baby's suckling action to help the milk to flow; however, the flow is typically not immediate, especially in the first 2 days, when the mother continues to make colostrum, the milk of the pregnancy hormones. Colostrum is thick, sticky, and rich in immunoglobulins. Because colostrum is so viscous, it is transferred more slowly.

When the same baby is suckling at the bottle, she is dealing with several differ-

---

[b] This term refers to the nipple in the case of the bottle or to the combination of nipple and breast tissue taken into the mouth during breastfeeding.

ent conditions, including: 1) the teat of the bottle is typically smaller and firmer than her mother's nipple and expands less in her mouth; 2) the teat delivers milk continuously from the beginning of the feed; and 3) infant formula is less viscous than colostrum, creating another difference in the fluid flow. Since these feeding methods are somewhat different, one can see that offering both methods could complicate the learning phase for many babies.

In North America, pacifiers and bottles are considered synonymous with infancy. The general public is largely unaware of the negative impact these devices may have on breastfeeding. Prenatal education and broader community education may be needed to raise awareness of these issues. In addition, parents need assistance in identifying other methods for soothing infants.

■ Expectations Regarding Artificial Teat Use

Maternity care staff should avoid routine introduction of artificial teats (bottle nipples and pacifiers) to healthy, full-term breastfeeding infants. When a healthy term infant requires supplementation, it should be administered in a way that limits potential future breastfeeding problems. The preferred methods for administering needed supplements would be via cup or a supplemental feeding device used at the breast. See Box 9-1 for more information.

There may be a role for pacifier use with the preterm infant who cannot yet be fed by mouth. The rationale for this is that the act of suckling causes the release of gastric hormones that foster the growth of the baby's gastrointestinal tract.[8]

Box 9-1   Feeding Devices

At-breast feeders:
- Baby gets additional milk while at the breast through a tube attached to reservoir.
- Mother's body gets the message to make more milk while baby is getting additional milk from the supplemental feeding device.
- Hospitals often use syringes with feeding tubes attached.

Cup feeding:
- Cups are inexpensive, available, and easy to clean.

- Growing body of research indicates the safety and efficacy for both term and preterm infants.
- Baby sets his or her own pace.
- When cup feeding, sit the baby upright. Do not pour the milk into the baby's mouth. Tip the cup slightly so that the milk is at the edge of the cup. Rest the cup gently on the baby's lower lip. The baby may sip, slurp, or lap milk from the cup.

Spoon feeding:
- We like to use small plastic spoons to collect drops of expressed colostrum if needed in the first few days.

In the event that a parent requests that his or her healthy, full-term infant receives a bottle or pacifier, staff should explore the reasons for this request with the parents, in order to foster informed decision making.

■ Evidence

The Effects of Exposure to Bottles on Breastfeeding Outcomes

Several studies identify an association between the use of bottles and subsequent breastfeeding difficulty. Righard reported on a group of 51 Swedish mother/infant pairs experiencing difficulties with breastfeeding technique. Compared with 40 control pairs without problems, bottle and pacifier use was significantly higher among the pairs with feeding difficulty.[9]

Howard, Howard, Lanphear, Eberly, de-Blieck, Oakes, et al. examined the impact of supplements delivered via bottle and cup on subsequent breastfeeding outcomes, finding that supplemental feedings delivered by either method had a detrimental effect on the continuation and subsequent exclusivity of breastfeeding.[10] However, when infants were born via cesarean delivery, and when infants required more than two supplements during their hospital stay, using a cup to deliver the supplement was less detrimental to ongoing breastfeeding than was bottle feeding.

The Effects of Pacifiers on Breastfeeding

In addition to studying the impact of bottles on breastfeeding duration and exclusivity, Howard et al. also examined the effect of pacifier use on the same outcomes.[11] Infants

in the study population were randomized to introduce pacifiers at 2–5 days of life or after 4 weeks of age. The infants in the early pacifier group were less likely to be exclusively breastfeeding at 4 weeks of age and had a shorter overall duration of breastfeeding.

Kramer, Barr, Dagenais, Yang, Jones, Cofani, et al. reported on a double blind randomized, controlled trial of 281 Canadian infants in which one group received a recommendation to use pacifiers beginning in the hospital and one group did not.[12] Parents who did not receive the pacifier recommendation received other suggestions for calming upset infants. The experimental intervention had no statistically significant impact on weaning at 3 months; however, a strong association between pacifier use and early weaning was observed. The authors mention that their data strongly suggest that pacifier use may be a marker of decreased comfort or mother's motivation to breastfeed and possibly of an existing breastfeeding difficulty. This same conclusion has been reached by other research teams.[13–15]

The impact of pacifiers on breastfeeding outcomes may not be immediately visible in the breastfed infant. Soares, Giugliani, Braun, Salgado, de Oliveira and de Aguiar reported that nearly 66% of pacifier users had ceased exclusive breastfeeding by 2 months of age, compared with 45% of nonpacifier users.[16] Righard and Alade found that 94% of pacifier use in their study population began before 2 weeks postpartum and occurred before breastfeeding problems were reported.[17] In babies who used pacifiers for greater than 2 hours per day, breastfeeding problems were more prevalent than among those who used pacifiers for less time or not at all. Ninety-one percent of mother/baby couplets who did not use pacifiers were breastfeeding at 4 months of age, as compared with 44% of pacifier users. Thus, research indicates that pacifier use, especially for greater than 2 hours per day, may be an indicator of both breastfeeding difficulties and increased risk of early weaning. This finding has been reported by other research teams.[18,19]

Victora, Behague, Barros, and Olinto report on a Brazilian study that had both qualitative and quantitative arms.[20] Echoing research reported previously, they found that infants who used pacifiers intensely were four times more likely than nonusers to have stopped breastfeeding by 6 months of age. During the ethnographic portion of this study, they found that many of the women who strongly encouraged pacifier use were ambivalent or unconfident about breastfeeding, and many of those used the pacifier to get the child off the breast or to increase the interval between feedings. The researchers state, "The latter also had rigid breastfeeding styles that increased maternal-infant distance, had important concerns about objective aspects of infant growth and development, and were highly sensitive to infant crying. These behaviors were linked to intense comparison between themselves and other mothers and to a lack of self-confidence."[21] The authors state that these women need help to face the challenges of breastfeeding and to build confidence in their ability to nourish their babies. It follows from this that mothers who request pacifiers for their babies during the maternity stay may be indicating a lack of confidence in their ability to breastfeed or physical, mental, or emotional discomfort with breastfeeding. Exploring why they are asking for pacifiers

may open the door to greater understanding and opportunities for support and education.

Routine early pacifier use has increased recently in response to research linking pacifier use with a reduction in sudden infant death syndrome (SIDS). At this time, the research seems to indicate that SIDS deaths are lower among populations of babies who use pacifiers during sleep periods. Hauck, Omojokun, and Siadaty published a meta-analysis on this topic and found evidence that in the United States one SIDS death could be prevented for every 2733 infants who used a pacifier when put to sleep.[22] Due to the concern about negative influence of early pacifier use on breastfeeding outcomes, as well as the rare occurrence of SIDS in the first weeks of life, the authors affirm: "For breastfed infants, pacifiers should be introduced after breastfeeding has been well established, which is consistent with the AAP policy statement on breastfeeding. Because SIDS is less common in the first month of life, it is reasonable to delay pacifier introduction during this lower risk period."[23]

A challenge of interpreting research on this topic is that most studies are retrospective case analyses or case/cohort analyses. There are currently no available prospective controlled trials on the topic, which makes causation difficult to prove. It should be noted that SIDS rates are significantly lower among breastfed infants,[24] and they are influenced by a myriad of other factors, including prenatal and postpartum household smoking, sleeping position, entanglement/entrapment issues related to the sleep environment, cosleeping issues, brain stem maturation, and many other causes.[25] Use of a pacifier cannot prevent SIDS, but it may reduce the risk of SIDS deaths. The risk for SIDS death appears greater for infants who routinely suckle on a pacifier at bedtime if they do not have the pacifier at a particular sleep time. This means that care must be taken to continually offer pacifiers if the infant is habituated to use one. However, many authorities indicate that parents should not reinsert their baby's pacifier if it falls out of the baby's mouth during sleep.

Researchers have proposed several possible mechanisms by which pacifier use might decrease SIDS deaths, including positioning the tongue forward and thus protecting the airway, increasing arousability in the infant, reduction in gastroesophageal reflux and aspiration, presence of the pacifier in the mouth making it less likely that the baby will move around and be covered by blankets or roll over to a prone sleeping position, among others.[26]

Along with several other recommendations to decrease the risk of SIDS death, AAP's task force on sudden infant death syndrome recommends that parents "consider offering a pacifier at nap time and bedtime . . . *For breastfed infants, delay pacifier introduction until 1 month of age to ensure that breastfeeding is firmly established* [italics added]."[27]

Other concerns have been expressed about pacifiers, including the increased risk of ear infection in children who use pacifiers habitually.[28] For this reason, AAP recommends that pacifier use be reserved for sleep times only and cease by the end of the first year.

Evidence Regarding the Safety of Bottle-Feeding

Bottle-feeding has long been a standard of infant feeding. Because the use of the bottle predates the current trend of evidence-based medicine, the safety of the bottle as an infant feeding device has not been well explored.

The only body of literature on the safety of bottle-feeding that can be located easily on Medline pertains to the feeding of preterm infants. In this special population, Marinelli, Burke, and Dodd monitored premature infants' heart rates, oxygen saturation rates, and respiratory rates during cup feeding and bottle-feeding, finding heart rates lower and oxygen saturation higher during cup feeding.[29] There were no statistical differences in respiratory rates or the occurrence of choking, spitting up, or apnea between the two methods. The authors concluded that cup feeding was an acceptable supplementation method for preterm infants.

Limited research in term infants also indicates that infants at the breast have lower heart and respiratory rates and higher oxygen saturation when breastfed than when receiving supplements via the bottle or cup. This indicates that breastfeeding is the least energy-consuming option—thus bottles or cups should not be administered with a rationale that it takes less work to feed via these methods. This suggests that feeding at the breast takes less energy than the bottle and cup, as homeostasis is better maintained.

Evidence Regarding the Safety of Cup Feeding

Cup feeding is the preferred method of supplementation of the World Health Organization and UNICEF. The rationale for using the cup is both to decrease the impact of the bottle teat, as well as to provide a safe, available supplementation device that can be easily cleaned. Cups are found in nearly every household, and their cleanliness can be easily ascertained. Bottles and teats are more difficult to clean and require special cleaning brushes for adequate care.

A recent Cochrane review on cup feeding concluded that use of the cup as a supplemental feeding device was significantly associated with increased probability of full breastfeeding at the time of hospital discharge, but no statistically significant correlation was found with maintaining full breastfeeding at 3 and 6 months postdischarge.[30] In addition, one study included in the Cochrane review found that cup feeding was associated with increased risk of prolonged hospital stay. Additional large-scale research is needed to quantify the effects of different supplementation methods.

The Howard study discussed previously identified that supplementation via cup as well as bottle methods were potentially detrimental to the continuation of breastfeeding, although the authors identified a decreased impact of the cup versus the bottle when the baby was born via cesarean delivery and when the baby required multiple supplements.[31]

Evidence Regarding Other Supplemental Feeding Methods

Common alternative feeding methods used during the postpartum stay include gastric tube (typically only inserted for infants with a medical need for repeated supplementation and for whom suckling is not an option), at-breast supplementers, finger feeding using a tube device, and spoon and dropper feeding. There is scant research evidence about the safety and outcomes of these methods.

A Medline search revealed no studies looking at the effects of supplements delivered via gastric tubing through the nose or mouth on breastfeeding outcomes. Similarly, no studies regarding use of spoons or droppers as supplemental feeding devices were identified.

At-breast supplementers use a fine tube to deliver expressed breast milk or formula to the baby as it suckles at the breast. No studies of the use of these devices were found in a recent Medline search.

Some lactation specialists use a feeding tube attached to the mother's or caregiver's finger in a feeding method called finger feeding. A Medline search identified only one study looking at the outcomes of finger feeding. Oddy and Glenn report on implementation of finger feeding as the chief supplementation method in the special care nursery during a hospital's work to achieve Baby-Friendly hospital designation.[32] Data indicated that 44% of infants were breastfeeding at discharge prior to and 71% were breastfeeding at discharge after implementation of the finger feeding method of supplementation. The authors report that the finger feeding technique was used to correct the sucking technique of the baby. However, as other hospital policies and practices undoubtedly changed during the process of becoming Baby-Friendly, it is difficult to know to what extent the method of supplementation played a role in breastfeeding outcomes. In addition, this data pertains to the preterm infant. The outcomes of research on finger feeding in a full-term population are currently unpublished.

In its protocol for supplementation of the breastfed infant, the Academy of Breastfeeding Medicine states:

> When supplemental feedings are needed, one of the following techniques may be used: a supplemental nursing device at breast, cup feeding,

spoon or dropper feeding, finger-feeding, or bottle feeding. There is little evidence about the safety or efficacy of most alternative feeding methods and their effect on breast-feeding; however, when cleanliness or refrigeration is sub-optimal, cup feeding may be the best choice. Cup feeding has been shown to be safe for term infants and may help preserve breast-feeding duration among those that require multiple supplemental feedings.[33]

■ Overcoming Common Barriers to Reducing Exposure to Artificial Teats

One of the most difficult barriers to reducing artificial teat exposure is the *cultural assumption that artificial teats are a normal part of infant care.* Parents and health providers alike typically share this assumption. In traditional cultures, a baby is likely to be carried in a soft sling against the mother's body, where the rhythmic motion of the mother's body and the reassuring sound of her heartbeat and voice soothe the baby. In modern Western culture, babies are often expected to remain quiet and be self-sufficient between regularly scheduled feedings. Many parents seem to expect that babies will sleep for most of the day, and all of the night! They can be overwhelmed by the thought that babies need very frequent interaction with their caregivers and may resort to using pacifiers and bottles to calm babies down when they are seeking contact and attention.

To counteract this barrier, it is best to first educate staff (see also Chapter 2) about the comfort needs of infants and the ideal avoidance of artificial teats in the learning phase of breastfeeding. Staff members may need guidance in learning how to teach methods of infant soothing that they can teach to parents. The most basic and powerful soothing method is skin-to-skin contact between the baby and one of its parents. Skin-to-skin contact is a powerful strategy that is often used only in the first hours after birth, although its power continues throughout infancy. If skin-to-skin contact is not helpful, then parents should be encouraged to walk or rock with their babies, to speak or sing soothingly to the baby, to change baby's diaper, and to observe for any pain baby may be experiencing. The breast or expressed breast milk should always be offered before considering administering a bottle or pacifier (unless, of course, medical conditions indicate immediate need for additional supplementation—see Chapter 6).

While a bottle or pacifier may seem a quicker solution to resolving the baby's distress, it may begin a whole negative cascade of events that reinforce a mother's concern for the adequacy of her milk supply, and for her baby's desire to suckle at her breast. The mother's confidence should be considered a key factor in determining continuation of breastfeeding. Taveras, Capra, Braveman, Jensvold, Escobar, and Lieu found that mothers who expressed lack of confidence in their ability to breastfeed on day 1 or 2 after birth were more likely to discontinue breastfeeding by 2 weeks after birth.[34]

Supplemental Feeding Devices

While it is ideal to avoid introduction of the bottle teat to the breastfed newborn, *staff members are often unfamiliar with other methods of supplementation.* Education and training are needed so that staff members develop a sense of skill and competency in assisting families with these feeding methods.

It may help to begin education with a review of the literature around supplemental feeding devices, as well as the supplementation protocol of the Academy of Breastfeeding Medicine. Staff need to understand the rationale for avoiding bottle teats before change in practice will be welcomed. Maternity managers, clinical specialists, and/or the quality improvement team may wish to consider conducting a small scale trial of various supplementation methods and resultant outcomes. One of the problems with the use of supplemental feeding devices during the maternity stay is that the outcomes for breastfeeding are largely unseen by the hospital staff, as mothers rarely return or report long-term breastfeeding outcomes. So *staff may feel justified in the belief that giving bottles or pacifiers to breastfed babies causes no harm.* Collecting follow-up data from one's own population is sometimes the most expedient way of making any resultant problems visible to the members of the health system.

Implementation of prolonged skin-to-skin contact, self attached feedings, and rooming-in with gradual adopting of collaborative feedings during the hospital stay will promote a decreased need for supplementation of the breastfed infant. When babies have unfettered, around-the-clock access to their mothers, they are likely to suckle more frequently and transfer more milk.

In addition to developing skill in the use of supplemental feeding devices, staff need opportunities to practice how to reply to requests from parents to provide a pacifier or relief bottle. An experienced breastfeeding care provider can model a compassionate counseling technique for responding to these requests. Staff can then be offered the opportunity to role play these conversations with each other. It is crucial to explore the motivating factors behind each request. Perhaps the mother sincerely doubts the adequacy of her milk supply; perhaps she mistakenly believes that she must wait so many hours between feedings to allow her breasts to fill up or to teach the baby about schedules. Every request is an opportunity to listen to the inner concerns and beliefs and offer clarification, reassurance, and education as needed.

Certain staff members may exhibit *resistance to change* regarding supplementation and/or pacifiers. In this case, it may be helpful to lock up formula, bottles, nipples, and pacifiers and require that they are signed out, including identification of the staff member, the identity of the patient, and the reason for use of the item. This action both assists in identifying who is using the items most often (thus identifying individuals needing further education and support), as well as effectively limiting unnecessary use. Some institutions have gone so far as to place pacifiers, formula, and bottles within the hospital's Pyxis or other computerized automated systems for administering drugs, thus reducing access to these items while simultaneously streamlining data collection regarding common users of these items.

Resources

Cordes, R., Howard, C. R., & Wight, N., for the Academy of Breastfeeding Medicine. (2002). Protocol #3: Hospital guidelines for the use of supplementary feedings in the healthy term breastfed neonate. New Rochelle, NY: Academy of Breastfeeding

Medicine. Available at http://bfmed.org/ace -images/ProtocolSuppl3rev.pdf.

Task Force on Sudden Infant Death Syndrome, AAP. (2005). The changing concept of sudden infant death syndrome: Diagnostic coding shifts, controversies regarding the sleeping environment, and new variables to consider in reducing risk. *Pediatrics, 116,* 1245–1255.

References

1. Neifert, M., Lawrence, R. A., & Seacat, J. (1995). Nipple confusion: Toward a formal definition. *The Journal of Pediatrics, 126,* S125–S129.

2. Fisher, C., & Inch, S. (1996). Nipple confusion— who is confused? *The Journal of Pediatrics, 129*(1), 174–175.

3. Woolridge, M. W. (1996). Problems of establishing lactation. *Food and Nutrition Bulletin, 17*(4). Retrieved November 7, 2007, from http://www. unu.edu/unupress/food/8F174e/8F174E06.htm.

4. Nowak, A. J., Smith, W. L., & Erenberg, A. (1994). Imaging evaluation of artificial nipples during bottle feeding. *Archives of Pediatric and Adolescent Medicine, 148,* 40–42.

5. Smith, W. L., Erenberg, A., & Nowak, A. (1988). Imaging evaluation of the human nipple during breast-feeding. *Archives of Pediatric and Adolescent Medicine, 142,* 76–78.

6. Mizuno, K., & Ueda, A. (2006). Changes in sucking performance from nonnutritive sucking to nutritive sucking during breast- and bottle-feeding. *Pediatric Research, 59*(5), 728–731.

7. Mathew, O. P. (1991). Science of bottle feeding. *The Journal of Pediatrics, 119*(4), 511–519.

8. Uvnas-Moberg, K. (1989). Gastrointestinal hormones in mother and infant. *Acta Paediatrica Scandinavica Supplement, 351,* 88–93.

9. Righard, L. (1998). Are breastfeeding problems related to incorrect breastfeeding technique and the use of bottles and pacifiers? *Lancet, 25*(1), 40–44.

10. Howard, C. R., Howard, F. M., Lanphear, B., Eberly, S., deBlieck, E. A., Oakes, D., et al. (2003). Randomized clinical trial of pacifier use and bottle-feeding or cupfeeding and their effect on breastfeeding. *Pediatrics, 111*(3), 511–518.

11. Howard, C. R., Howard, F. M., Lanphear, B., Eberly, S., deBlieck, E. A., Oakes, D., et al. (2003). Randomized clinical trial of pacifier use and bottle-feeding or cupfeeding and their effect on breastfeeding. *Pediatrics, 111*(3), 511–518.

12. Kramer, M. S., Barr R. G., Dagenais, S., Yang, H., Jones, P., Cofani, L., et al. (2001). Pacifier use, early weaning, and cry/fuss behavior: A randomized controlled trial. *Journal of the American Medical Association, 286*(3), 322–326.

13. Righard, L. (1998). Are breastfeeding problems related to incorrect breastfeeding technique and the use of bottles and pacifiers? *Lancet, 25*(1), 40–44.

14. Benis, M. M. (2002). Are pacifiers associated with early weaning from breastfeeding? *Advances in Neonatal Care, 2*(5), 259–266.

15. Ullah, S., & Griffiths, P. (2003). Does the use of pacifiers shorten breastfeeding duration in infants? *British Journal of Community Nursing, 8*(10), 458–463.

16. Soares, M. E., Giugliani, E. R., Braun, M. L., Salgado, A. C., de Oliveira, A. P., & de Aguiar, P. R. (2003). Uso de chupeta e sua relação com o desmame precoce em população de crianças nascidas em Hospital Amigo da Criança [Pacifier use and its relationship with early weaning in infants born in a Child-Friendly Hospital]. *Journal of Pediatrics (Rio J), 79*(4), 309–316.

17. Righard, L., & Alade, M. O. (1997). Breastfeeding and the use of pacifiers. *Birth, 24,* 116–120.

18. Victora, C. G., Tomasi, E., Olinto, M. T., & Barros, F. C. (1993). Use of pacifiers and breastfeeding duration. *Lancet, 341*(8842), 404–406.

19. Cunha, A. J., Leite, A. M., & Machado, M. M. (2005). Breastfeeding and pacifier use in Brazil. *Indian Journal of Pediatrics, 72*(3), 209–212.

20. Victora, C. G., Behague, D. P., Barros, F. C., & Olinto, M. T. (1997). Pacifier use and short breastfeeding duration: Cause, consequence or coincidence? *Pediatrics, 99*(3), 445–453.

21. Victora, C. G., Behague, D. P., Barros, F. C., & Olinto, M. T. (1997). Pacifier use and short breastfeeding duration: Cause, consequence or coincidence? *Pediatrics, 99*(3), 445.

22. Hauck, F. R., Omojokun, O. O., & Siadaty, M. S. (2005). Do pacifiers reduce the risk of sudden infant death syndrome? A meta-analysis. *Pediatrics, 116*(5), e716–e723. Available at http:// pediatrics.aappublications.org/cgi/reprint/116/5/ e716.

23. Hauck, F. R., Omojokun, O. O., & Siadaty, M. S. (2005). Do pacifiers reduce the risk of sudden infant death syndrome? A meta-analysis. *Pediatrics, 116*(5), e716–e723. Available at http:// pediatrics.aappublications.org/cgi/reprint/116/5/ e721.

24. Ip, S., Chung, M., Raman, G., Chew, P., Magula, N., DeVine, D., et al. (2007). Breastfeeding and maternal and infant health outcomes in developed countries. Evidence report/technology assessment No. 153 (Prepared by Tufts-New England Medical Center Evidence-based Practice Center, under Contract No. 290-02-0022). AHRQ Publication No. 07-E007. Rockville, MD: Agency for Healthcare Research and Quality. Available at http://www.ahrq.gov/clinic/tp/brfouttp.htm.

25. Task Force on Sudden Infant Death Syndrome and AAP. (2005). The changing concept of sudden infant death syndrome: Diagnostic coding shifts, controversies regarding the sleeping environment, and new variables to consider in reducing risk. *Pediatrics, 116,* 1245–1255.

26. Community Paediatrics Committee, Canadian Pediatric Society. (2003). Recommendations for the use of pacifiers. *Pediatrics & Child Health,* 8(8), 515–519. Retrieved November 7, 2007, from: http://www.cps.ca/english/statements/CP/cp03-01.htm.

27. Community Paediatrics Committee, Canadian Pediatric Society. (2003). Recommendations for the use of pacifiers. *Pediatrics & Child Health,* 8(8), 1252.

28. Niemela, M., Pihakari, O., Pokka, T., & Uhari, M. (2000). Pacifier as a risk factor for otitis media: A randomized, controlled trial of parental counseling. *Pediatrics, 106*(3), 483–488.

29. Marinelli, K. A., Burke, G. S., & Dodd, V. L. (2001). A comparison of the safety of cupfeedings and bottlefeedings in premature infants whose mothers intend to breastfeed. *Journal of Perinatology, 21*(6), 350–355.

30. Flint, A., New, K., & Davies, M. W. (2007). Cup feeding versus other forms of supplemental enteral feeding for newborn infants unable to fully breastfeed. *Cochrane Database of Systematic Reviews,* (2), CD005092.

31. Howard, C. R., Howard, F. M., Lanphear, B., Eberly, S., deBlieck, E. A., Oakes, D., et al. (2003). Randomized clinical trial of pacifier use and bottle-feeding or cupfeeding and their effect on breast-feeding. *Pediatrics, 111*(3), 511–518.

32. Oddy, W. H., & Glenn, K. (2003). Implementing the Baby-Friendly Hospital Initiative: The role of finger feeding. *Breastfeeding Review, 11*(1), 5–10.

33. Cordes, R., Howard, C. R., & Wight, N., for the Academy of Breastfeeding Medicine. (2002). Protocol #3: Hospital guidelines for the use of supplementary feedings in the healthy term breastfed neonate. New Rochelle, NY: Academy of Breastfeeding Medicine, p. 3. Retrieved November 7, 2007, from http://bfmed.org/ace-images/ProtocolSuppl3rev.pdf.

34. Taveras, E. M., Capra, A. M., Braveman, P. A., Jensvold, N. G., Escobar, G. J., & Lieu, T. A. (2003). Clinician support and psychosocial risk factors associated with breastfeeding discontinuation. *Pediatrics, 112*(1 Pt 1), 108–115.

Ten Steps to Successful Breastfeeding
A Joint WHO/UNICEF Statement[a]

Every facility providing maternity services and care for newborn infants should:

1. Have a written breastfeeding policy that is routinely communicated to all healthcare staff.
2. Train all healthcare staff in skills necessary to implement this policy.
3. Inform all pregnant women about the benefits and management of breastfeeding.
4. Help mothers initiate breastfeeding within a half-hour of birth. (US, one hour)
5. Show mothers how to breastfeed, and how to maintain lactation even if they should be separated from their infants.
6. Give newborn infants no food or drink other than breastmilk unless medically indicated.
7. Practice rooming in—allow mothers and infants to remain together—24 hours a day.
8. Encourage breastfeeding on demand.
9. Give no artificial teats (US, nipples) or pacifiers (also called dummies or soothers) to breastfeeding infants.
10. **Foster the establishment of breastfeeding support groups and refer mothers to them on discharge from the hospital or clinic.**

[a] World Health Organization. (1989). *Protecting, promoting and supporting breast-feeding: The special role of maternity services.* Geneva, Switzerland: World Health Organization, p. iv.

CHAPTER

10

Keeping Breastfeeding Going

Bridging the Gaps Into the Community

In maternity care facilities around the world, mothers and families gather together with other mothers, families, and their babies in living rooms, solariums, learning centers, and dining rooms. Parents chat informally with each other and attend parent education sessions during the maternity stay. In some settings, parent groups are formed by the childbirth educator, midwife, doula, or OB care provider. It's expected that parents who have babies around the same age will form informal, "friendship" and support groups.

Formal breastfeeding support groups are also found around the world; La Leche being the most notable. With leaders facilitating, these groups provide information, support, and social learning to new and experienced breastfeeding mothers. Peer counselors may also be part of maternity care and public health programs and are an effective strategy for promoting and supporting breastfeeding.

Baby cafés, community drop-in centers, usually funded with public health money, are becoming increasingly common. Located in public spaces, the café may change locations and time from day to day providing a facilitated local spot for pregnant women and mothers to meet, socialize, and learn from one another.

The vast majority of a successful breastfeeding experience goes on outside the walls of the maternity facility. However, what happens during the maternity stay has a profound long-term effect on feeding outcomes, including whether or not the staff provide linkage between the mother and breastfeeding resources outside the facility. All breastfeeding mothers will need additional support after their discharge. The maternity facility plays a key role in establishing optimal breastfeeding, identifying and addressing any breastfeeding issues that arise in the peripartum period, and assuring that women are encouraged to utilize existing support services in the community.

Research indicates that women continue to experience concerns and problems with breastfeeding for weeks and months after giving birth. However, the early weeks after birth are the most vulnerable time for unplanned weaning. Taveras, Capra, Braveman, Jensvold, Escobar, and Lieu found that 25% of the breastfeeding women in their sample stopped breastfeeding within the first 2 weeks and that 45% had stopped by 12 weeks.[1] The reasons women gave for weaning

varied with the age of baby. Discontinuation by 2 weeks was higher among women with little confidence in breastfeeding during the hospital stay. In addition, women cited early breastfeeding problems as a key reason for weaning by the second week. Discontinuing breastfeeding by week 12 was associated with maternal symptoms of depression and also with difficulty combining breastfeeding with return to work or school. Women who reported having received breastfeeding encouragement from a clinician were less likely to wean in the first 3 months. Thus, women may abandon breastfeeding if they do not receive the support and encouragement they deserve. During the hospital stay, it is crucial that hallmarks of potential future problems are identified and appropriately referred.

If breastfeeding is not optimally initiated during the maternity stay, problems can arise at home. Readmission for hyperbilirubinemia, hypernatremia, and/or dehydration has been documented as a sequelae of inadequate breastfeeding during the hospital stay and inadequate follow-up in the community. In 1995, Cooper, Atherton, Kahana, and Kotagal reported on a rising trend toward readmission of breastfed infants for hypernatremia, citing five cases admitted over a 5-month period to a Cincinnati tertiary care center with an average weight loss of 23% of body weight and elevated serum sodium levels.[2] The authors summarized:

> while breastfeeding malnutrition and hypernatremia is not a new problem, this cluster of infants represents an increase in frequency and severity of the problem and could be a consequence of several factors, including inadequate parent educa-

tion about breastfeeding problems and inadequate strategies for infant follow-up.[3]

In 2005, Moritz, Manole, Bogen, and Ayus reviewed all admissions of newborn infants to a children's hospital in Pittsburgh over a 5-year period, finding that 1.9% had breast-feeding-associated hypernatremia.[4] Mean weight loss in these infants was 13.7% at the time of admission. Most presented with visible jaundice. None of the babies were found to have bacteremia or meningitis. Most of the mothers were primiparae who were discharged within 48 hours of birth. They conclude: "Hypernatremic dehydration requiring hospitalization is common among breastfed neonates. Increased efforts are required to establish successful breastfeeding."[5]

To avoid problems such as hypernatremia, it is essential that mothers and babies learn excellent breastfeeding management techniques, including appropriate latch and attachment, as well as the importance of unrestricted feedings on the baby's cue. Infrequent and inadequate feeding is correlated with increased risk of hyperbilirubinemia.[6] Rather than being caused by breastfeeding, hypernatremia is caused by *inadequate* breastfeeding. Cadwell has proposed that a hospital's readmission rate for hyperbilirubinemia may be a marker of how well it is supporting mothers and babies in initiating breastfeeding.[7]

It is also essential that breastfed infants receive adequate follow-up in the community. The American Academy of Pediatrics has stated that feeding adequacy should be assessed by a pediatrician or other professional at 3 to 5 days of age, including physical examination for jaundice and hydration and a formal observation of breastfeeding,

followed by a second ambulatory visit at 2 to 3 weeks of age to monitor weight gain and provide support.[8]

Medical evaluation and encouragement is only one type of support that breastfeeding mothers need. Many women are unaware of other community resources for breastfeeding assistance such as La Leche League, Nursing Mothers Council, WIC programs, peer support programs, and breastfeeding care providers among others. Most mothers do not need highly technical support services; rather, most need assessment and reassurance (when appropriate). However, specialized services may be needed by those mother/baby couplets that did not get off to a good start, as well as by those who are working with physical or developmental issues that complicate breastfeeding, such as prematurity, prior breast surgery, or Down syndrome.

Communities in North America may provide breastfeeding support in many different sectors, including:

- Mother-to-mother breastfeeding support through voluntary agencies (La Leche League, Nursing Mothers Council, etc.)
- Professional breastfeeding support in the healthcare system (lactation support workers employed in pediatric/obstetric/family practice and midwifery offices; or hospital-based outpatient breastfeeding clinics and support groups, etc.)
- Breastfeeding support in the public health system (cross-training public health/visiting nurses; establishing breastfeeding support services within the WIC setting, including one-on-one counseling, groups, and breastfeeding education via professional staff or peer counselors, etc.)

- Breastfeeding support in child development programs (integrating breastfeeding into early parenting programs such as Zero to Three or Zero to Five programs, Early Headstart, and other regional and local community service programs that work to advance parent/child bonding and knowledge of child development).
- Breastfeeding support in communities of faith (offering breastfeeding support groups and services through Jewish Family Services, churches, mosques, etc.)
- Breastfeeding support in workplaces and schools (employer/school sponsored pumping rooms and breastfeeding counseling).

Expectations for Provision of Ongoing Support

All breastfeeding women should leave the hospital with knowledge of and linkage to available support in the community. Any woman who has experienced breastfeeding problems or had concerns about the adequacy of her milk supply should receive an individualized care plan prior to discharge, including a plan for professional follow-up as well as general support.

It is not enough for the maternity unit to distribute a list of available resources. Rather, staff on the postpartum unit should be intimately involved in the ongoing process of assessing the needs for and assuring the provision of ongoing support. Hospitals and birth centers may host breastfeeding support groups; invite groups in the community to hold meetings on facility property; or refer mothers to existing groups in the community.

Evidence for the Importance of Ongoing Breastfeeding Support

Common Pitfalls in the Early Postpartum Period

Lewallen, Dick, Flowers, Powell, Zickefoose, Wall, et al. followed several hundred women who began breastfeeding in the hospital, finding that more than 30% of women stopped breastfeeding prior to 8 weeks and another 37% were supplementing breastfeeding with formula at 8 weeks.[9] Insufficient milk was the most common reason cited by women for early weaning, followed by painful breasts/nipples, returning to work or school, and concerns about drugs or illness in the baby. The authors state: "The primary reasons for early cessation of breastfeeding are amenable to nursing intervention. Every opportunity should be taken to address these issues both in the hospital and through follow-up calls."[10] Most of the women in this study population reported that they received help with their concerns during the hospital stay, but only 55% reported receiving any help after discharge. These results are mirrored by those of many other studies, finding a quick drop-off in breastfeeding in the early weeks of breastfeeding and a lack of a system for providing breastfeeding support in most U.S. communities.

What Kind of Support Is Most Helpful to Women?

Britton, McCormick, Renfrew, Wade, and King conducted a Cochrane review of the effectiveness of postpartum support for breastfeeding mothers, finding that while both lay and professional support had a positive effect on breastfeeding duration, lay support appeared more effective at increasing exclusive breastfeeding, and professional support was more effective at increasing the duration of any breastfeeding.[11]

Postpartum support need not be offered in a one-on-one style. A recent study from Singapore examined the outcomes of a two-session postpartum lactation support program including a visit by a lactation specialist during the hospital stay with a second session at 1 to 2 weeks postdelivery, finding that the women in the support program had increased incidence of any breastfeeding and of exclusive breastfeeding at 2 weeks, 6 weeks, 3 months, and 6 months compared to the control group.[12] The researchers calculated that in order to achieve a goal of one woman exclusively breastfeeding at 6 months, 11 women would need to be treated via the postnatal support program tested.

Guise and colleagues conducted a systematic review of the effectiveness of research studies originating in the primary care setting for the U.S. Preventive Services Task Force (also discussed in Chapter 3).[13] Educational programs were found to have the greatest effect of any single intervention on both initiation and short-term duration of breastfeeding. Support offered via telephone, in person, or both increased the duration of breastfeeding. Distribution of pamphlets and other written materials was not found to significantly increase breastfeeding.

Having examined the data about breastfeeding support offered outside the hospital setting, de Oliveira, Camacho, and Tedstone confirmed the need to combine multiple strategies to assist the mother in achieving her breastfeeding goals.[14]

The Pregnancy Risk Assessment Monitoring System, a data system used in many states in the United States, assesses the maternal experiences, behaviors, and attitudes before, during, and after pregnancy. The survey includes an opportunity for new mothers across the nation to make free text comments on their experience. A recent report analyzed womens' responses, finding the six major themes, of which the top three are pertinent to this discussion: (1) need for social support, (2) breastfeeding issues, and (3) lack of education about newborn care after discharge.[15]

■ Common Barriers to Providing Ongoing Support and Strategies to Overcome Them

One barrier to providing ongoing support is the *fragmentation of the health system* in the United States. Unless the maternity unit is part of a health maintenance organization, the providers of prenatal, postpartum, and pediatric care in the community may have little interaction with the maternity facility staff. Similarly, the ancillary breastfeeding support system may not be integrated into the health system in a way that fosters good communication among caregivers. The result of this lack of coordinated communication means that mothers and babies with problems may fall between the cracks, not receiving appropriate referral and follow-up.

Working to establish a lactation referral system can help in closing gaps in service. For an example of this work in action, see Box 10-1.

Box 10-1 Case in Point: Developing a Breastfeeding Referral System

One local community awoke to the gaps in its lactation support system when a baby was rehospitalized after a loss of more than 25% of its body weight. The baby was suffering from hypernatremic dehydration secondary to insufficient milk supply caused by prior breast reduction surgery. While the baby did not suffer long-term effects of this experience, it awoke the medical and support community to the problem of gaps in service. A task force was formed to review the case and make a recommendation on how to avoid such outcomes in the future.

The task force identified that the obstetric care provider had documented the history of breast reduction surgery, which had occurred 5 years prior to the birth of this baby. The obstetric records indicated that the mother had reported the occurrence of the surgery, had stated an intention to breastfeed, and had a history of breastfeeding her two older children, who were born prior to the reduction surgery.

The breast reduction surgery was not noted in the prenatal records that were forwarded to the hospital. Hospital records did not indicate that history of breast surgery was discussed during the hospital stay. Hospital records indicated that the baby lost 9% of birth weight during the stay, and that breastfeeding was assessed. Nursing staff had documented visible evidence of colostrum and one meconium bowel movement in the 46 hours prior to discharge. The mother and baby were discharged to the community. Although the mother had requested a public health nurse visit, she did not receive priority for a visit due to her multiparity.

Pediatric records indicated that the mother had spoken with a nurse at the pediatric office twice regarding concerns about the baby's sleepiness. Routine pediatric care was scheduled by the office to occur at 1 month of age. However, the baby was seen by the pediatric care provider at 3 weeks, when the mother called to report that the baby was sleeping more than 5 hours at a stretch, falling asleep during feeds, and that she could no longer easily awaken the baby to feed. At the 3-week visit, the pediatrician immediately hospitalized the baby for symptoms of dehydration.

The review team found that several factors contributed to the outcome of dehydration:

- There was a lack of communication of the mother's history of breast surgery from the obstetrics provider to the hospital staff
- There was a lack of breast history taken during the hospital stay, as well as an inadequate breastfeeding assessment.
- Assumptions about the lactation ability of the mother were made on the basis of prior breastfeeding history without awareness of the potential impact of the reduction surgery.
- The baby did not have a timely routine pediatric assessment. The schedule of pediatric assessment in the community was not in compliance with AAP policy.
- There was a lack of communication between the obstetric and pediatric offices of the history of breast reduction surgery in the mother.

In order to decrease chances of occurrence of this problem, the review team recommended that a communitywide breastfeeding referral

/continues

Box 10-1 **Case in Point: Developing a Breastfeeding Referral System (continued)**

system be developed. A task force was created with representation from the pediatric, inpatient, obstetric, public health, and lactation specialist communities. The task force drafted and piloted a referral form to be used by any care provider in the community to identify existing risk factors for breastfeeding problems present in the prenatal period as well as to communicate the existence of problems or issues in the postpartum period. The form was produced in carbonless duplicate form, so that copies could be distributed to pertinent care providers.

Prenatal risk factors included history of breast surgery, presence of inverted nipples, routine use of medications of concern for breastfeeding safety, etc. The prenatal care provider would use the referral form to communicate the presence of a risk factor to both the hospital and the pediatric care provider. As a matter of practicality, the hospital would receive both the hospital and pediatric copies of the form and forward the pediatric form on to the family's chosen pediatric care provider

with an update on progress on the issue during the hospital stay.

Postpartum risk factors include the existence of maternal concern about adequacy of milk supply, mastitis, feeding difficulty in the baby, etc. Any care provider consulting with the mother and/or baby during the postpartum period could use the form to communicate the existence of problems and follow-up strategies to others in the community. After testing and refining the form, it was widely distributed throughout the care provider community and used with satisfaction by several care providers. A need for an annual in-service meeting on the use of the tool was identified after a few years of use. In this way, providers were reminded of the existence of this valuable tool, and input was gathered on how to refine the tool with provider feedback

The Moral of the Story: Working together, a community can develop a system designed to tighten existing gaps in providing continuity of care.

In acknowledgment of the challenges of ongoing breastfeeding, the maternity facility should work with community partners to establish a solid support network for breastfeeding families. Community partners may include WIC programs, La Leche League, and Nursing Mothers Council groups, lactation support services and providers, pediatric, obstetric, midwifery, and family practice providers, parenting programs, Early Headstart, and other community resources for parents with young children. Working in collabora-

tion, these individuals and agencies can take inventory of the existing support services, identifying which support needs are well met and which are not adequately met. For example, many communities provide breastfeeding support groups during morning hours, but few during evening hours, thus not serving the needs of many mothers in the workforce. The maternity unit can work with its collaborators to explore methods of meeting this and other unmet needs. See Box 10-2 for an illustration of how a hospital and

WIC program might work together to solve support needs.

Another barrier is *lack of awareness of limitations or availability of resources.* Many units

---

Box 10-2 **An Example of Hospital–Community Collaboration to Provide Breastfeeding Support**

Mothers' Milk Forever Hospital (MMFH) serves three rural counties, comprising more than 300 square miles of mountainous terrain. When MMFH's breastfeeding task force met with the local WIC breastfeeding coordinator to assess community breastfeeding support, they were unable to identify any local breastfeeding support groups. There were no existing La Leche League or Nursing Mothers Council groups within 750 miles of their hospital. The only lactation specialists in the area were an International Board Certified Lactation Consultant (IBCLC) who worked at MMFH and a breastfeeding counselor who worked for WIC. Both WIC and the hospital had tried independently to establish breastfeeding support groups. However, attendance at the groups was low, especially in the winter months when traveling many miles to the hospital over snowy roads was difficult. The MMFH and WIC staff put their heads together to try to identify an appropriate solution to their area's particular needs. They decided to explore a peer counseling model by identifying successful breastfeeding women in key locations throughout their catchment area who would agree to be trained as peer counselors. The WIC coordinator was able to secure peer counselor training funds, and the hospital was able to provide space and refreshments for the training, which was conducted in keeping with the state WIC peer counseling training program.

Once trained, the 10 peer counseling graduates accepted referrals of pregnant women from the

WIC program and postpartum women from the hospital. Most of the peer counselors provided telephone support to the women assigned to them. The peer counselors who lived close to the hospital began to make rounds with the hospital's IBCLC and, with her guidance, learned to provide bedside support and teaching to the mothers. Some of the other peer counselors who lived close to outlying WIC clinics began attending during clinic hours and prenatal classes in order to meet pregnant and postpartum clients and share some of their own breastfeeding experiences. In this way, the skill and competency of the peer counselors grew. Some of the peer counselors began to hold support groups in more heavily populated areas, using church halls and community centers as their locations. Over time, a wide network of activities grew from the energy of the peer counselors, including breastfeeding booths at the annual agricultural fair, a breastfeeding-is-welcome-here program for local businesses, and the establishment of several long-term breastfeeding support groups. This collaboration between the hospital and WIC resulted in much higher rates of breastfeeding continuation in the community, as well as the establishment of ongoing breastfeeding as a norm of parenting young children.

The Moral of the Story: Working together results in new and creative strategies to solve complicated problems.

distribute resource listings that are not up to date. Staff may be unaware of restrictions of resources, such as the inability of most WIC programs to provide services and breast pumps for women who do not meet income eligibility requirements.

One way to strengthen networking between and among breastfeeding resources is to establish a local or regional breastfeeding coalition. Through regular interaction, care providers can become more aware of the resources, limitations, and specialties of the organizations and individuals providing lactation care in the local community. Many communities have breastfeeding coalitions that meet in face-to-face format on a periodic basis, sometimes providing continuing education credits for presentations given as an incentive to attend meetings. Other areas have electronic discussion groups for lactation support that helps providers find resources for specific cases as well as providing a forum for announcing new support groups, changes to support offerings, etc.

Another barrier to ongoing support is *the difficulty of providing proactive resources.* Proactivity refers to the action of reaching out to those in need, rather than providing service in reaction to a request. It is relatively rare for mothers to reach out to unfamiliar resources for help. Rather, they will turn to their family or friends, who may or may not give accurate breastfeeding information and support. Often breastfeeding questions arise when the baby is difficult to soothe in the middle of the night. Even women who have just delivered a baby and are well aware that hospitals are staffed around the clock will refrain from calling the maternity unit for help. It is much more effective to reach out

to women, but it is difficult to operationalize and fund such proactive services.

Many hospitals have developed creative strategies for low-cost proactive solutions. Examples include:

- inviting La Leche League leaders or WIC breastfeeding counselors to hold breastfeeding groups in the maternity unit
- identifying the hospital staff who make follow-up calls to hospital patients to conduct surveys for marketing purposes and cross-train them to ask questions about breastfeeding progress and identify if mothers are connected with postpartum resources, providing referral to support services as needed
- having maternity nursing staff make follow-up calls to recently delivered mothers during downtime on the unit
- developing breastfeeding peer counseling programs to provide proactive contact with mothers in the community
- establishing breastfeeding drop-in centers where mothers are likely to be found—in the mall, at the pediatric clinic, etc.

Without connection to community care providers, maternity units can only provide limited support services after discharge. In order to secure ongoing breastfeeding, it is essential that the facility participate in building and maintaining solid connection with community resources.

References

1. Taveras, E. M., Capra, A. M., Braveman, P. A., Jensvold, N. G., Escobar, G. J., & Lieu, T. A., et al. (2003). Clinician support and psychosocial risk factors associated with breastfeeding discontinuation. *Pediatrics, 112*(1 Pt 1), 108–115.

2. Cooper, W. O., Atherton, H. D., Kahana, M., & Kotagal, U. R. (1995). Increased incidence of severe breastfeeding malnutrition and hypernatremia in a metropolitan area. *Pediatrics, 96*(5 Pt 1), 957–960.

3. Cooper, W. O., Atherton, H. D., Kahana, M., & Kotagal, U. R. (1995). Increased incidence of severe breastfeeding malnutrition and hypernatremia in a metropolitan area. *Pediatrics, 96*(5 Pt 1), 957.

4. Moritz, M. L., Manole, M. D., Bogen, D. L., & Ayus, J. C. (2005). Breastfeeding-associated hypernatremia: Are we missing the diagnosis? *Pediatrics, 116*(3), e343–e347.

5. Moritz, M. L., Manole, M. D., Bogen, D. L., & Ayus, J. C. (2005). Breastfeeding-associated hypernatremia: Are we missing the diagnosis? *Pediatrics, 116*(3), e343.

6. DeCarvalho, M., Klaus, M. H., & Merkatz, R. B. (1982). Frequency of breast-feeding and serum bilirubin concentration. *American Journal of Diseases of Children, 136*, 737–738.

7. Cadwell, K. (1998). Bilirubin status as an outcome measure in monitoring adherence to baby-friendly breastfeeding policies in hospitals and birth centers in the United States. *Journal of Human Lactation, 14*(3), 187–189.

8. AAP Section on Breastfeeding. (2005). Breastfeeding and the use of human milk. *Pediatrics, 115,* 499.

9. Lewallen, L. P., Dick, M. J., Flowers, J., Powell, W., Zickefoose, K. T., Wall, Y. G., et al. (2006). Breastfeeding support and early cessation. *Journal of Obstetric, Gynecologic, and Neonatal Nursing, 35*(2), 166–172.

10. Lewallen, L. P., Dick, M. J., Flowers, J., Powell, W., Zickefoose, K. T., Wall, Y. G., et al. (2006). Breastfeeding support and early cessation. *Journal of Obstetric, Gynecologic, and Neonatal Nursing, 35*(2), 166.

11. Britton, C., McCormick, F. M., Renfrew, M. J., Wade, A., King, S. E. (2007). Support for breastfeeding mothers. *Cochrane Database of Systematic Reviews,* (1), CD001141.

12. Su, L. L., Chong, Y. S., Chan, Y. H., Chan, Y. S., Fok, D., Tun, K. T., et al. (2007). Antenatal education and postnatal support strategies for improving rates of exclusive breast feeding: Randomised controlled trial. *British Medical Journal, 335*(7620), 596.

13. Guise, J. M., Palda, V., Westhoff, C., Chan, B. K., Helfand, M., & Lieu, T. A., for the U.S. Preventive Services Task Force. (2003). The effectiveness of primary care-based interventions to promote breastfeeding: Systematic evidence review and meta-analysis for the U.S. Preventive Services Task Force. *Annals of Family Medicine, 1*(2), 70–78.

14. de Oliveira, M. I., Camacho, L. A., & Tedstone, A. E. (2001). Extending breastfeeding duration through primary care: A systematic review of prenatal and postnatal interventions. *Journal of Human Lactation, 17*(4), 326–343.

15. Kanotra, S., D'Angelo, D., Phares, T. M., Morrow, B., Barfield, W. D., & Lansky, A. (2007, Nov.). Challenges faced by new mothers in the early postpartum period: An analysis of comment data from the 2000 Pregnancy Risk Assessment Monitoring System (PRAMS) survey. *Maternal and Child Health Journal, 11*(6), 549–558.

CHAPTER 11

The Baby-Friendly Hospital Initiative

A Tool for Change[a]

The Baby-Friendly Hospital Initiative (BFHI) is a proven platform for achieving continuity of care in the maternity setting regardless of demographics, annual number of births, acuity, provider mix, or culture of the patient population. As an organized accessible resource, the BFHI program and tools encourage the staff to progress toward measurable continuity of care practices within an evidence based structure. Receipt of the prestigious international WHO/UNICEF award after an

---

[a] This chapter contains material written by Cindy Turner-Maffei and originally published in 2002 as "Using the Baby-Friendly Hospital Initiative to Drive Positive Change." In Cadwell K. (Ed.). *Reclaiming Breastfeeding for the United States: Protection, Promotion, and Support,* pp. 23–33. Sudbury, MA: Jones & Bartlett Publishers. The material has been revised and updated.

on-site assessment and evaluation celebrates your achievement. On-going monitoring assures continued excellent care.

The Baby-Friendly Hospital Initiative is an international program that links breastfeeding with current American healthcare themes of quality improvement, evidence-based practice, and family-centered care. Created in 1991 by the World Health Organization (WHO) and the United Nations Children's Fund (UNICEF), the Baby-Friendly Hospital Initiative recognizes hospitals and birth centers that have fully implemented the *Ten Steps to Successful Breastfeeding,* which were first published in 1989 by UNICEF and WHO[1] (see Box 1-8). The initiative was inspired by the *Innocenti Declaration,*[2] the summary statement of the 1990 international policymakers' conference that listed four operational targets to be implemented worldwide, including the practice of the *Ten Steps to Successful Breastfeeding* by all maternity hospitals and centers.

The initiative also incorporates another target of the *Innocenti Declaration* by monitoring compliance of participating hospitals and birth centers with the *International Code of Marketing of Breastmilk Substitutes* (also known as the *International Code).*[3] This code covers all items used to replace breast milk in the first 6 months of life and includes infant formula and other infant foods marketed for babies under 6 months of age, as well as bottles, teats, and pacifiers. To comply with the *International Code,* hospitals accept no free or low-cost formula, teats, bottles, and pacifiers. Birth facilities comply with the *International Code* when they refrain from inadvertently advertising breast milk substitutes via visual presence of formula and formula feeding items in plain view of patients and staff, as well as via posters, signs, and visible formula product names

and logos. Code-compliant facilities do not distribute formula samples, gifts bearing logos and product names of replacement feeding items, or educational/marketing materials bearing product names and logos.

As of 2006, there were nearly 20,000 designated Baby-Friendly hospitals and maternity centers throughout the world. Comparatively, the United States had designated 62 of its hospitals and birth centers by the end of 2007. In addition, as of that date, 70 facilities in the United States participated in the initiative through the Certificate of Intent program. Roughly 3000 hospitals and birth centers in the United States are eligible for the award.

At the time of publication, there were nine designated Baby-Friendly hospitals in Canada.[4]

■ Baby-Friendly USA

In the United States, the Baby-Friendly Hospital Initiative is administered by Baby-Friendly USA, a nonprofit organization. In 1997, the United States Committee for UNICEF announced its partnership with the Healthy Children Project, Inc. in the creation of Baby-Friendly USA.[5] Implementation of the Baby-Friendly Hospital Initiative in the United States was the subject of a feasibility study conducted by an expert work group convened by the National Healthy Mothers, Healthy Babies coalition with support from the United States Department of Health and Human Services.[6] The expert work group was convened in 1992 and completed its deliberations in 1994. During that time, the United States Committee for UNICEF and consultant Minda Lazarov kept the U.S. initiative alive by creating the Certificate of Intent program through which hospitals and birth centers could register their intention to pursue designation. Wellstart International developed evaluation guidelines, criteria, and assessment tools for the U.S. initiative and piloted the 1996 assessment of Evergreen Medical Center of Kirkland, Washington, which was the first U.S. birth facility to receive the Baby-Friendly designation.

The philosophic touchstones of the U.S. Baby-Friendly Hospital Initiative are objective, inclusive, accessible, voluntary, and celebratory, which are explained as follows.

Objective: The initiative is based upon objective on-site assessment of compliance with the *Ten Steps to Successful Breastfeeding.*

Inclusive: All hospitals with maternity facilities as well as freestanding birth centers may participate in the initiative.

Accessible: Information and technical assistance is available to all participating facilities.

Voluntary: Birth facilities seek out and implement this program on their own, rather than having change forced upon them.

Celebratory: Baby-Friendly USA celebrates the achievements of facilities and gives positive reinforcement to those along the path of optimizing breastfeeding practices.

The goals of the Baby-Friendly Hospital Initiative are convergent with findings of several United States maternal health documents and campaigns. A description of these documents follows.

Recommendations of the 1984 Surgeon General's Workshop on Breastfeeding and Human Lactation:[7]

Improve professional education about human lactation and breastfeeding.

Develop public education and promotional efforts.

Strengthen the support for breastfeeding in the healthcare system.

Develop a broad range of support services in the community.

The U.S. Department of Agriculture's 1996 *Nutrition Action Themes*[8]

(5.1) Build multisectoral partnerships with a commitment to build a social culture supportive of breastfeeding.
(5.2) Regularly update nutrition components of established programs.
(5.3) Use state-of-the-art methods and technology.
(5.4) Expand proven interventions to fully reach the target groups.
(5.5) Improve policy action through research.

Call to Action: Better Nutrition for Mothers, Children, and Families[9]

(11.1) Promote breastfeeding as the preferred method of infant feeding.
(11.2) Continue efforts to develop more effective strategies to promote breastfeeding through hospitals, MCH, WIC, etc.
(11.3) Explore ways to promote breastfeeding through community efforts.
(11.5) Assure that healthcare professionals who interact with pregnant women ... communicate breastfeeding as the norm.
(11.8) Provide lactation management training to all healthcare professionals who interact with pregnant and breastfeeding women to enhance their ability to support breastfeeding, and involve hospitals in networking for the promotion of breastfeeding.

HHS Blueprint for Action on Breastfeeding[10]

This policy document recommends that the following steps be taken by the healthcare system...

• Establish hospital and maternity center practices that promote breastfeeding, such as the "Ten Steps to Successful Breastfeeding."

Breastfeeding in the United States: A National Agenda[11]

The United States Breastfeeding Committee developed this document, which identifies targets to achieve 4 major goals. Strategy 2 for the health system is "to ensure that every facility providing maternity services will offer effective, evidence-based breastfeeding care."[12] Under this strategy, the following activities are identified: "a) to encourage the USBC member organizations to promote best hospital practices to their members such as those identified in the WHO/UNICEF Baby-Friendly Hospital Initiative; b) Encourage the U.S. Department of Health and Human Services [DHHS] to issue a statement urging all maternity care facilities to provide effective, evidence-based breastfeeding practices such as those identified in the WHO/UNICEF Baby-Friendly Hospital Initiative."[13]

The Healthy People 2010 Goals[14]

(16-19) Increase the proportion of mothers who breastfeed their babies.

Objective	Increase in Mothers who Breastfeed	1998 Baseline	2010 Target
16-19a	In early postpartum period	64%	75%
16-19b	At 6 months	29%	50%
16-19c	At 1 year	16%	25%

In 2005, additional targets were added for exclusive breastfeeding. The targets as well as baseline data from 2004 follow:

		2004 Baseline	2010 Target
16-19d	Exclusive breastfeeding to 3 months	31%	40%
16-19e	Exclusive breastfeeding to 6 months	11%	17%

■ Using the Baby-Friendly Hospital Initiative to Effect Change

Data available from the 2004 National Immunization Survey[15] indicates the national average for breastfeeding was 73.8% at discharge from the hospital, while 41.5% continued to breastfeed at 6 months and 20.9% at 12 months, with exclusive breastfeeding rates at 30.5% at 3 months and 11.3% at 6 months. Comparatively, among women from families participating for the WIC program, the rates were 66.9% initiation, while 33.1% breastfed to 6 months and 16.7% to 12 months, with exclusive breastfeeding rates at 23.4% at 3 months, and 8.1% at 6 months. Women eligible to participate in the WIC program are of low and moderate income, and are among those least likely to initiate and continue breastfeeding their babies. Ironically, breastfeeding rates are lowest today among those families who could most benefit from the positive health, nutrition, economic, and empowerment outcomes of breastfeeding.

Factors influencing women's choices regarding breastfeeding are myriad. Preconceptual and prenatal breastfeeding promotion activities need to be carefully tailored to the concerns women express. However, even those women who choose or are persuaded to choose breastfeeding may be dissuaded by negative events during the peripartum period. One study of a WIC population reported that 68% of women interviewed prenatally planned to breastfeed exclusively, yet only 20% of these women were actually breastfeeding exclusively upon discharge from the hospital, and only 17% exclusively breastfed at home.[16] The experiences a woman has during the sensitive period around the time of birth have great ramifications upon her subsequent breastfeeding activities.[17]

The potential impact of the hospital environment on breastfeeding is brought into sharp focus by the *WIC Infant Feeding Practices Study*:

> Mothers experience a variety of circumstances in the hospital that are unsupportive of the establishment of breastfeeding. Something other than breastmilk as the first feeding, delayed timing of first breastfeeding, lack of rooming-in arrangements and hospital gift packages that contain formula, bottle, or a pacifier, are examples of

neonatal circumstances that may be unsupportive of the establishment of breastfeeding. Only twenty-nine percent of WIC mothers give their infants breastmilk as the first feeding. Sixty percent of WIC infants receive formula as the first feeding and 10 percent receive either sugar water or plain water.... Seventy-two percent of WIC infants sleep away from their mothers at least for one night during their hospital stay. Ninety-three percent of WIC mothers receive a gift package from the hospital. The gift packages of almost all WIC mothers contain items that are detrimental to the establishment of breastfeeding, such as formula, a bottle, or a pacifier. Among the mothers who receive a gift package, 86 percent get some formula in the package.... (T)hree quarters of breastfeeding mothers experience one or more nursing problems while they are still in the hospital. However, 33 percent of the mothers who experience nursing problems in the hospital receive no help from the hospital staff.[18]

These results are diametrically opposed to the Healthy People goals. The Healthy People goals include targets to reduce the economic, racial, and ethnic disparities in breastfeeding. WIC participants represent a diversity of low- and moderate-income families. Breastfeeding rates are lowest in these populations. It is truly unfortunate that the breastfeeding intentions of these mothers are often negatively influenced by outdated practices. Often the negative effect of practices is not visible to maternity staff who rarely have contact with mothers after discharge and therefore may have no knowledge of negative outcomes.

Mothers learn how to interact with their babies through the modeling behavior of maternity staff; this is particularly important for mothers' management of breastfeeding. The research of Reiff and Essock-Vital indicates that "Learning through modeling was more effective in shaping mothers' early infant-feeding choices than learning through verbal teaching."[19] Therefore, maternity staff must be aware that potential effects of actions may be greater still than those of words.

All of the negative practices identified in the WIC infant feeding practices excerpted previously articulate with the *Ten Steps to Successful Breastfeeding*. Therefore, the Baby-Friendly Hospital Initiative provides a platform for examining and improving breastfeeding policies, practices, and experiences. The *Ten Steps to Successful Breastfeeding* are supported by a body of research demonstrating the positive impact of each step.[20–23] Because this material comes from the World Health Organization and UNICEF, esteemed international sources, it may be regarded with more respect than initiatives originating from lesser known or more local or politicized sources.

■ The Journey Toward Baby-Friendly Designation

Hospitals and birth centers often begin the successful journey toward Baby-Friendly[24] designation by establishing a multidisciplinary team including representation from administration, marketing, quality improvement, and women's health services as well as medical and nursing staff members. The team may then request an information packet from the Baby-Friendly USA office.[b] Team members may review and complete the hospital self-appraisal tool included with the packet. Thorough, honest completion of this form identifies both those areas where the facility is already doing well with breastfeeding and highlights areas of weakness. Reviewing the tool together also provides opportunities for exploration of the beliefs and opinions of team members; often teams report that their initial meetings are largely focused on educating themselves about current breastfeeding practices and literature.

Once the tool is completed, it is recommended that the team celebrate the breastfeeding strengths of the facility. Next, the team prioritizes the areas of challenge from those easiest to accomplish or most fundamental to those most difficult or esoteric. The team then begins to establish a plan for the completion of the easiest steps first, working up to the most difficult. For example, many facilities find that steps such as rewriting policies, improving staff and patient education, and implementing evidence-based practices are much easier targets to tackle than are other steps such as the establishment of a business relationship with the formula vendors including the purchase of formula or removing pacifiers from well-baby units. Once stronger policies are established, staff and patients are better educated about breastfeeding, practices

---

[b] Baby-Friendly USA, 327 Quaker Meeting House Road, E. Sandwich, MA 02537. Telephone: (508) 888-8044. Email: www.babyfriendlyusa.org. Readers outside the United States should contact their national authority for the BFHI. The web site www.babyfriendly.org offers linkage to the home pages of the initiative in many countries.

such as skin-to-skin contact are routinely implemented and the breastfeeding rate soars, which may surprise team members and staff. With a much smaller percentage of mothers choosing formula for their babies, the price tag of formula purchase is markedly decreased. *Overcoming Barriers to Implementing the Ten Steps to Successful Breastfeeding* addresses strategies that have been used to overcome this and other barriers to successful implementation of the *Ten Steps to Successful Breastfeeding.*[25]

Physician and administrative involvement has been crucial to success in many facilities. Writing of Boston Medical Center's journey, Merewood and Philipp state, "We have come to the conclusion that physician leadership, or at the very least physician commitment to the Baby-Friendly venture, was and is critical to success."[26]

Many facilities have found it beneficial to focus on the quality improvement aspects of the initiative; seeing breastfeeding through the quality healthcare lens helps to clarify the health and practice implications described more fully in Chapter 13. Every facility that receives accreditation through the Joint Commission on Accreditation of Healthcare Organizations (JCAHO) knows the value of voluntary quality improvement processes.

Hospitals have become interested in the role that women play in guiding the healthcare choices and decisions of family members and developed women's health centers and specialties to focus on meeting the needs of women. The Baby-Friendly Hospital Initiative has great potential to provide high quality, proactive care for women at a vulnerable time of their lives, the birth and nourishment of a new baby. Meeting women's needs well during this crucial time period may forge a lasting, positive perception of the healthcare facility and personnel.

Facilities wishing to pursue Baby-Friendly designation first apply for a certificate of intent. Certificate of Intent hospitals receive technical assistance from Baby-Friendly USA staff as well as the opportunity to participate in on-line discussion groups of staff at other maternity care facilities who are working on the initiative or who have achieved the award. Later, following consultation with Baby-Friendly USA staff, participating facilities may request an on-site assessment. This assessment includes interviews with mothers, staff, and administrators, review of documents, and observations of mothers and staff. Findings of the assessment team are forwarded to the external review board consisting of representative experts from across the nation, who consider the assessment findings and make a determination regarding designation of the Baby-Friendly award. Facilities not designated upon first assessment and external review are encouraged to request reassessment once the identified remaining challenges are overcome.

■ Evaluation of Implementation of the *Ten Steps to Successful Breastfeeding*

How well are maternity facilities doing at implementing the *Ten Steps to Successful Breastfeeding*? Several small-scale studies have looked at this question.[27,28] Assessing Philadelphia area hospitals, Kovach found that these hospitals were only partially implementing the four steps she identifies as key: breastfeeding initiation, staff education, supplementation, and rooming-in.[29] Dodgson,

Allard-Hale, Bramscher, Brown, and Duckett studied Minnesota hospitals and found that adherence was highest (39%) for step 4 (help mothers initiate breastfeeding within an hour of birth), and lowest for steps 1 (have a written breastfeeding policy), 9 (give no artificial teats or pacifiers), and 10 (foster the establishment of breastfeeding support groups). Steps 1, 9, and 10 were adhered to at 2.4%, 4.9%, and 0% of the hospitals, respectively.[30]

A study from researchers at the Centers for Disease Control and the Food and Drug Administration identifies the synergistic effect of the *Ten Steps to Successful Breastfeeding*.[31] Using data from the federal infant feeding practices study, the researchers were able to identify the level of exposure to five of the *Ten Steps to Successful Breastfeeding* among 1100 women participating in the longitudinal survey who chose to breastfeed their infants. Only 7% of mothers interviewed experienced care in line with all five steps measured. Compared with mothers who experienced all five steps, mothers who experienced no steps were eight times more likely to stop breastfeeding early. The risk factors most strongly associated with early weaning were late breastfeeding initiation and supplementation of the infant. The authors state:

> These results suggest that the cumulative effect of these practices, rather than each individual practice, is most important in breastfeeding outcome. In addition, the fact that a very small percentage of women (7%) reported experiencing all five of the Baby-Friendly practices measured in this study illustrates the need to increase efforts aimed at implementing these

strategies within the hospital environment.[32]

Clark and Deutsch of Kaiser Permanente's Moanalua Medical Center of Honolulu, Hawaii, the second U.S. Baby-Friendly Hospital, shared their hospital's experience of the Baby-Friendly process in a 1997 article.[33] They cited several strategies for their successful organizational change, including the development of an interdisciplinary team, a prioritized work plan, and early implementation of staff education. Education, policy, and teamwork were the cornerstones of their journey. The next step was identification of indicators of success. Indicators were measured and assessed regularly, and results were used to make continuous improvements. Emphasis was placed on involving all players, sharing the plan, staying focused on the vision, and celebrating all achievements.[34]

■ The Impact of Implementation of the Baby-Friendly Hospital Initiative

Statistics from around the world indicate the positive outcomes associated with successful implementation of the *Ten Steps to Successful Breastfeeding*. In China, after 2 years of BFHI implementation, exclusive breastfeeding rates doubled in rural areas and increased from 10% to 47% in urban areas.[35] In Cuba, exclusive breastfeeding rose from 25% in 1990 to 72% in 1996.[36]

The PROBIT study, a large randomized trial conducted in the former Soviet Republic of Belarus, has provided insight into the potential child health benefits of implementation of the *Ten Steps to Successful Breastfeeding*.[37] Prior to the study, hospitals and polyclinics, the health centers through which all citizens receive their health care, practiced maternity procedures similar to those practiced in Western communities in the 1970s and 1980s. This difference allows for "greater potential contrast between intervention and control study sites. However, Belarus resembles Western developed countries in one very important respect: basic health services and sanitary conditions are very similar."[38] The study protocol randomized hospitals and polyclinics to two groups; in the intervention group, extensive staff training was undertaken to implement the 10 steps, while in the control group facilities, no changes were made to breastfeeding practices or protocols. Information about the infants born during the years of the study was collected in all visits to the polyclinic for pediatric care. Data was collected for more than 17,000 mother/infant pairs. Compared to infants born at the control sites, infants born at the intervention sites were significantly more likely to be breastfed to any degree at 12 months and to be breastfed exclusively at 3 months and at 6 months. Infants born in the intervention sites had a significant reduction in the risk of gastrointestinal tract infections and atopic eczema, but no significant reduction in respiratory tract infection. The authors conclude: "These results provide a solid scientific underpinning for future interventions to promote breastfeeding."[39]

Merten, Dratva, and Ackermann-Liebrich reported on breastfeeding practices among a random sample of more than 3000 Swiss women delivering in 145 hospitals throughout the country.[40] They found that although breastfeeding rates improved throughout the population, breastfeeding duration was significantly longer among mothers who had given birth in Baby-Friendly hospitals with a high degree of compliance with the *Ten Steps to Successful Breastfeeding*. The authors conclude that the increase in breastfeeding rates in Switzerland since 1994 is partially due to the increasing number of Baby-Friendly birth facilities in the country.

A before-and-after study from Turkey also demonstrates a significant increase in breastfeeding duration into the second year of life after implementation of the BFHI, finding that overall breastfeeding duration rates increased by 1.5 times after implementation of the 10 steps.[41] The long-term effects of improved practice in the maternity setting are significant, indeed! What happens during the maternity stay has long-term consequences for the future of breastfeeding, and thus the health of the population.

Data collected in 2001 from the first 28 U.S. hospitals and birth centers to achieve the Baby-Friendly designation showed a mean breastfeeding initiation rate of 83.8%, compared with an overall U.S. breastfeeding initiation rate of 69.5% in that same year.[42] Exclusive breastfeeding rates at the same facilities averaged 78.4%, compared with a national mean of 46.3%. The researchers noted that demographic characteristics typically associated with lower breastfeeding rates were not associated with lower rates in the Baby-Friendly facilities. This finding suggests that changing hospital policy and practice can improve the playing field for breastfeeding success.

■ Benefits of Participation in the Baby-Friendly Hospital Initiative

Clark and Deutsch found that the benefits of the Baby-Friendly Hospital fell into three categories: improved care and service to members; utilization of resources; and positive public image. "For us, it has never been about the award or recognition. It's about healthy babies who can grow to be healthy children in nurturing families. It's about a philosophy of care—an attitude communicated by caregivers in an environment of love, assistance, and encouragement."[43]

Facilities participating in the initiative can reap benefits such as team building; quality improvement; health promotion (with resultant cost savings to healthcare systems and insurers); customer satisfaction; and local, national, and international recognition of achievement. Through their work to implement the *Ten Steps to Successful Breastfeeding,* hospitals and birth centers strive to meet the needs of each new mother and baby with state-of-the-art care that does not interfere in the development of the breastfeeding relationship, thereby assisting in the growth of stronger, healthier families and communities.

References

1. World Health Organization and United Nations Children's Fund. (1989). *Protecting, promoting and supporting breast-feeding: The special role of maternity services.* Geneva, Switzerland: WHO.
2. United Nations Children's Fund. (1990). *Innocenti declaration on the protection, promotion and support of breastfeeding.* Florence, Italy, and New York: UNICEF.
3. World Health Organization. (1981). *International code of marketing of breast-milk substitutes.* Geneva, Switzerland: WHO.
4. The Breastfeeding Committee for Canada. (2007). *Baby-Friendly hospitals and birthing centers in Canada.* Retrieved February 25, 2008 from http://breastfeedingcanada.ca/pdf/BCC%20List%20of%20Designated%20Facilities%20January%202008.pdf.
5. U.S. Committee for UNICEF. (1997). *U.S. infants at risk of suffering lifelong chronic illnesses.* New York: Author.
6. Lazarov, M., Feldman, A., & Silveus, S. (1993). The Baby Friendly Hospital Initiative: US activities. *Journal of Human Lactation, 9*(2), 74.
7. Spisak, S., & Gross, S. S. (1991). *Second followup report: The surgeon general's workshop on breastfeeding and human lactation.* Washington, DC: National Center for Education in Maternal and Child Health.
8. U.S. Department of Agriculture. (1996). *Nutrition action themes for the United States: A report in response to the International Conference on Nutrition* [CNPP-2]. Washington, DC: Author.
9. Sharbaugh, C. O. (Ed.). (1990). *Call to action: Better nutrition for mother, children, and families.* Washington, DC: National Center for Education in Maternal and Child Health.
10. U.S. Department of Health and Human Services. (2000). *HHS Blueprint for Action on Breastfeeding.* Washington, D.C: U.S. Department of Health and Human Services, Office on Women's Health, p. 19.
11. United States Breastfeeding Committee. (2001). *Breastfeeding in the United States: A national agenda.* Rockville, MD: U.S. Department of Health and Human Services, Health Resources and Services Administration, Maternal and Child Health Bureau.
12. United States Breastfeeding Committee. (2001). *Breastfeeding in the United States: A national agenda.* Rockville, MD: U.S. Department of Health and Human Services, Health Resources and Services Administration, Maternal and Child Health Bureau. p. 7.
13. United States Breastfeeding Committee. (2001). *Breastfeeding in the United States: A national agenda.* Rockville, MD: U.S. Department of Health and Human Services, Health Resources and Services Administration, Maternal and Child Health Bureau. p. 8.
14. U.S. Department of Health and Human Services. (2000, January). *Healthy People 2010—Conference edition.* Washington, DC: Author.
15. Centers for Disease Control and Prevention. (n.d.). Table 1. Breastfeeding Rates by Socio-demographic

Factors, Among Children Born in 2004. Retrieved on 2/25/08 at http://www.cdc.gov/breastfeeding/data/NIS_data/2004/socio-demographic.htm.

16. Romero-Gwynn, E. & Carias, L. (1989). Breast-feeding intentions and practice among Hispanic mothers in southern California. *Pediatrics, 84*(4), 626.

17. Jelliffe, D. B., & Jelliffe, E. F. P. (1988). *Programmes to promote breastfeeding.* New York: Oxford Press.

18. Baydar, N., McCann, M., Williams, R., Vesper, E., & McKinney, P. (1997, November). Final Report: WIC Infant Feeding Practices Study. Washington, DC: United States Department of Agriculture, Food and Nutrition Service, Office of Analysis and Evaluation. Contract No. 53-3198-3-003, pp. 5–6.

19. Reiff, M. I., & Essock-Vitale, S. M. (1985). Hospital influences on early infant-feeding practices. *Pediatrics, 76*(6), 872.

20. World Health Organization. (1998). *Evidence for the Ten Steps to Successful Breastfeeding* [WHO/CHD/98.9]. Geneva, Switzerland: Author.

21. Powers, N. G., Naylor, A. J., & Wester, R. A. (1994). Hospital policies: Crucial to breastfeeding success. *Seminars in Perinatology, 18*(6), 517.

22. Perez-Escamilla, R., Pollitt, E., Lönnerdal, B., & Dewey, K. G. (1994). Infant feeding policies in maternity wards and their effect on breast-feeding success: An analytic overview. *American Journal of Public Health, 1,* 89.

23. Saadeh, R. & Akre, J. (1996). Ten steps to successful breastfeeding: A summary of the rationale and scientific evidence. *Birth, 2 3,* 154.

24. In the United States, the terms "Baby-Friendly" and "Baby-Friendly Hospital Initiative" are trademarks of the U.S. Fund for UNICEF.

25. Turner-Maffei, C., & Cadwell, K., eds. (2004). *Overcoming Barriers to Implementing the Ten Steps to Successful Breastfeeding.* Sandwich, MA: Baby-Friendly USA. Available at http://www.babyfriendlyusa.org/eng/docs/BFUSAreport.pdf.

26. Merewood, A., & Philipp, B. L. (2001). Implementing change: Becoming Baby-Friendly in an inner city hospital. *Birth, 28,* 36.

27. Karra, M. V., Auerbach, K. G., Olson, L., & Binghay, E. P. (1993). Hospital infant feeding practices in metropolitan Chicago: An evaluation of five of the 'Ten Steps to Successful Breastfeeding.' *Journal of the American Dietetic Association, 93*(12), 1437.

28. Wright, A., Rice, S., & Wells, S. (1996). Changing hospital practices to increase the duration of breastfeeding. *Pediatrics, 97*(5), 669.

29. Kovach, A. C. (1997). Hospital breastfeeding policies in the Philadelphia area: A comparison with the *Ten Steps to Successful Breastfeeding. Birth, 24*(1), 41.

30. Dodgson, J. E., Allard-Hale, C. J., Bramscher, A., Brown, F., & Duckett, L. (1999). Adherence to the ten steps of the Baby-Friendly Hospital Initiative in Minnesota hospitals. *Birth, 26*(4), 239.

31. DiGirolamo, A. M., Grummer-Strawn, L. M., & Fein, S. (2001). Maternity care practices: Implications for breastfeeding. *Birth, 28,* 94.

32. DiGirolamo, A. M., Grummer-Strawn, L. M., & Fein, S. (2001). Maternity care practices: Implications for breastfeeding. *Birth, 28,* 98.

33. Clark, L. L., & Deutsch, M. J. (1997). Becoming Baby-Friendly. *AWHONN Lifelines, 12,* 30.

34. Clark, L. L., & Deutsch, M. J. (1997). Becoming Baby-Friendly. *AWHONN Lifelines, 12,* 34.

35. UNICEF Programme Division. (1999). *Baby-Friendly Hospital Initiative: Case studies and progress report.* New York: Author.

36. UNICEF Programme Division. (1999). *Baby-Friendly Hospital Initiative: Case studies and progress report.* New York: Author.

37. Kramer, M. S., Chalmers, B., Hodnett, E. D., Sevkovskaya, Z., Dzikovich, I., Shapiro, S., et al. (2001). Promotion of breastfeeding intervention trial (PROBIT): A randomized trial in the Republic of Belarus. *Journal of the American Medical Association, 285,* 413.

38. Kramer, M. S., Chalmers, B., Hodnett, E. D., Sevkovskaya, Z., Dzikovich, I., Shapiro, S., et al. (2001). Promotion of breastfeeding intervention trial (PROBIT): A randomized trial in the Republic of Belarus. *Journal of the American Medical Association, 285,* 413.

39. Kramer, M. S., Chalmers, B., Hodnett, E. D., Sevkovskaya, Z., Dzikovich, I., Shapiro, S., et al. (2001). Promotion of breastfeeding intervention trial (PROBIT): A randomized trial in the Republic of Belarus. *Journal of the American Medical Association, 285,* 413.

40. Merten, S., Dratva, J., & Ackermann-Liebrich., U. (2005, November). Do Baby-Friendly Hospitals influence breastfeeding duration on a national level? *Pediatrics, 116*(5), e702–e708.

41. Duyan Camurdan, A., Ozkan, S., Yüksel, D., Pasli, F., Sahin, F., & Beyazova, U. (2007). The effect of the Baby-Friendly hospital initiative on long-term breast feeding. *International Journal of Clinical Practice, 61*(8), 1251–1255.

42. Merewood, A., Mehta, S. D., Chamberlain, L. B., Philipp, B. L., & Bauchner, H. (2005). Breastfeeding rates in US Baby-Friendly hospitals: Results of a national survey. *Pediatrics, 116*(3), 628–634.

43. Clark, L. L., & Deutsch, M. J. (1997). Becoming Baby-Friendly. *AWHONN Lifelines, 12,* 37.

CHAPTER

12

Providing Woman-Centered Breastfeeding Care^a

As we have discussed throughout this book, maternity care policies and practices have a great effect on breastfeeding outcomes. This book has explored the importance of policy, staff training, perinatal education, early and continuous skin-to-skin contact, unrestricted breastfeeding guided by skilled caregivers, avoidance of unnecessary supplements, continuous rooming-in, unrestricted breastfeeding, avoidance of artificial teats and pacifiers, and linkage to ongoing breastfeeding support as cornerstones of establishing the breastfeeding experience. However, good practice governs not only *what* is done, but also *how* it is done. This

^a This chapter contains material adapted from an article written by Cynthia Turner-Maffei & Karin Cadwell, originally published in March 2007 as "What Do Breastfeeding Women Want?" *eBreast*. Available at http://nursing.jbpub.com/ezine/.

chapter will explore the qualitative aspects of breastfeeding care that have been found beneficial in assisting the mother and baby in attaining comfortable, effective, confident breastfeeding practices.

Every mother giving birth is a unique person, as is every baby, every father, every support person, and every member of the healthcare team. In trying to understand the experience of the individual family through the lens of accumulated experience, caregivers may lose focus on each family's unique reality. One example is a mother with sore nipples on the second postpartum day. One approach to helping her might be to think of the last several mothers who had sore nipples and apply solutions that worked in a majority of those cases. While this can be helpful in generating lists of potential solutions, it does not help the caregiver to understand the unique experience of the mother who presents with the complaint of sore nipples. A different approach might be to seek to discover what *this* mother's experience of sore nipples has been and how she would like to be helped.

Counseling skills are at the root of discovering this information. Many health professionals have little or no formal training in counseling. Yet, it is a core skill of lactation care. See Table 12-1 for more information.

■ What Do We Know About How Women Want to Be Helped by Their Caregivers?

A growing body of qualitative research offers insight into women's experiences of being helped with breastfeeding. Raisler[1] found that mothers described as *helpful* those care providers who:

- Knew correct information
- Established supportive personal relationships
- Referred women to breastfeeding specialists for problems
- Showed enthusiasm for breastfeeding
- Facilitated breastfeeding through concrete interactions during the childbearing period

Women participating in Raisler's research identified as *unhelpful* those care providers who:

- Missed opportunities to discuss breastfeeding
- Gave misinformation
- Encouraged formula supplementation
- Provided perfunctory or routine breastfeeding care
- Were hard to contact when problems arose

Several qualitative studies encourage care providers to think differently about how to give lactation care. Common threads of many research studies indicate that women seek the following:

- Ownership of decision making regarding infant feeding
- Psychosocial support during labor
- Continuity of care during the postpartum stay
- Consistency of information
- Companionable presence at a full feeding
- Individualized feeding assessment
- Hands-off teaching
- Individualized education
- A woman-centered approach
- Emotional and concrete support

Table 12-1   Key Components of Mother-Centered Counseling

Activity	Counseling Component	Example
Create a comfortable environment	• Introduce yourself • Ask open-ended questions • Establish equality by sitting or standing at the same level	*Nurse:* **"Hello Ms. Fielding. My name is Fatima. I'm your nurse this shift. May I sit with you for a few minutes?"** *Mother:* "Yes, certainly. Call me Jessica, please." N: **"Thank you Jessica! How are you and baby Joe doing today?"** M: "I'm doing well, but I'm worried about Joe. He hasn't eaten for a while."
Explore the mother's concerns	• Accept the concerns or questions she raises (whether you agree with them or not) • Use reflective listening to explore her concerns in greater depth • Adopt a level of language that echoes the mothers' (e.g., "pee and poop" rather than "urination and bowel movements") • Deal with her concerns in an empathetic, low-key manner so that the mother senses respect and may gain reassurance	N: **"Aah, I see. You are concerned that Joe may not be feeding enough and is quite sleepy?"** M: "Yes. The last time he ate was more than 6 hours ago, and he's been asleep since then." N: **"Tell me more. Let's see, he was born about 12 hours ago, right? What were the first feedings like?"** M: "Wonderful. He latched right on the first time and suckled a lot. But then he got quite sleepy. He nursed one other time after that, then we both slept for a while." N: **"So he's had 2 feedings since he was born? And how about dirty diapers? Have you changed any?"** M: "The first nurse changed one after each feeding. He had peed and pooped some of that awful green stuff both times." N: **"So Joe has had two pees and poops. That's good news. You seem to be very aware of Joe's habits. That's great."** M: "I want to be a good mother. I've dreamed of having a baby and breastfeeding for years. I'm so worried it won't work out." N: [Makes empathetic sounds] **"It all seems a little overwhelming right now, but maybe Joe can help us."**

/continues

Table 12-1 **Key Components of Mother-Centered Counseling (continued)**

Activity	Counseling Component	Example
Guide the development of mothering skills	• Ask permission to change the scenario • Reinforce the mother's and baby's instinctive behavior • Reinforce the importance of mother/baby unity • Teach signs of feeding readiness and milk transfer	N: *"I notice that he is moving around a bit in the bassinet. May I pick him up and bring him closer to you?"* M: *"Yes."* N: *"Babies just love to be held skin-to-skin by their parents. They seem to wake up more easily when they are skin-to-skin. May I unwrap Joe so he can snuggle with you?"* M: *"OK. But won't he get cold?"* N: *"There's no warmer place for him than in your arms. Let's tuck him under your gown . . . there. Look at that smile. He sure knows his momma!"* M: *"Hello, baby boy!"* N: *"How happy he is to be with you. Look at that smile!"* M: *"Wow! What's he doing? Is he trying to feed on his own?"* N: *"You are right, look at that! He sure knows what he wants! Hurrah, Joe!"* M: *"So he knows when he wants to feed? I don't have to worry about the time between feedings?"* N: *"As long as he's close to you, skin to skin, he will let you know when he's ready to feed. When he's all bundled up in a separate bed, he may have a harder time showing you when he wants to feed."* M: *"So when he starts hunting around for the nipple, it's time to feed?"* N: *"Yes. Also, when he starts moving his hand toward his mouth, or rolling his eyes under the lids, or making little mouthing movements."* M: *"Oh, he does those things often."* N: *"That's good! Well, when he does those things, help him come to the breast. You can know that he wants milk, and you have it ready for him! Listen to him swallowing! Oh, and now he's pooping! These are good signs that he is getting milk."* M: *"What a smart boy I have!"* N: *"Together, you are a great team!"*

/continues

Table 12-1	Key Components of Mother-Centered Counseling (continued)	
Activity	**Counseling Component**	**Example**
Plan for future interactions	• Determine what type of additional help the mother would like	M: "Well it seems like he's done now." N: **"Yes. What else is on your mind?"** M: "I'd really like to go to the bathroom. Would you sit with him for a minute while I go?" N: **"Of course."** M: [Coming back]. "Thanks for your help. I feel better now that he fed and pooped." N: **"What would you like to do now?"** M: "I think I'd like to take a nap. Could you push the bassinet over here so I can keep him close to me in case he needs me?" N: **"Certainly … here's my pager number. Please call me when you wake up, and we'll chat some more, OK?"** M: "Sounds good. Thank you!"

Ownership of Decision Making Regarding Infant Feeding

Many women do not appreciate care that seems to dictate their behavior. Hoddinott and Pill state, "Women were keen to maintain ownership, control, and responsibility for their own decision-making about infant feeding."[2] While it is important for maternal staff to explore and inform women's feeding decisions, it is crucial that staff members recall that the parents must make the best decision for themselves. Once introduced to the potential ramifications of infant feeding choices, it can be difficult for some healthcare workers to refrain from judgment regarding parents' individual decisions.

Respectful care should always be given, regardless of infant feeding choices. Infant feeding counseling training is essential in developing the ability of staff members to explore decision making in a respectful manner.

Psychosocial Support During Labor

Multiple studies have demonstrated the powerful effects of psychosocial support, or doula care, during the peripartum period. Langer, Campero, Garcia, and Reynoso demonstrated a significantly higher rate of exclusive breastfeeding 1 month after birth after doula-supported labor.[3]

Continuity of Care During the Postpartum Stay

Ekström and Nissen observed the effect of continuous support offered by midwives and nurses with special breastfeeding counseling training, finding that the intervention strengthened the maternal relationship with the baby and the mother's feelings for the baby.[4]

Consistency of Information

A major complaint made by postnatal women is that the healthcare staff give inconsistent and sometimes contradictory information and advice. Staff training and ongoing staff dialogue can help build collaboration and reduce inconsistency.[5]

Companionable Presence at a Full Feeding

Gill found that mothers expected nurses to stay with them during an entire feeding, especially the first feeding.[6] This is not an unreasonable expectation—as humans we learn few other motor skills without assistance throughout the first attempts. (Imagine a swimming lesson where the instructor walked away once the student entered the pool!) Yet, this can be difficult to operationalize in healthcare settings where bedside staff are responsible for several mother/baby couplets simultaneously. Few hospitals employ an adequate number of lactation specialists to allow full feeding evaluation for every mother/baby pair—indeed this might be a misuse of the time of the lactation specialist. All bedside nursing staff in the maternity unit should be able to coach a mother through her initial feeds. See Chapter 5 for strategies employed by many facilities to allow feeding observation of multiple mother/baby pairs simultaneously.

Individualized Feeding Assessment

In their exploration of the impact of health systems factors on breastfeeding, Kuan, Britto, Decolongon, Schoettker, Atherton, and Kotagal found that mothers reported the most helpful interaction to be individualized feeding assessment conducted by a hospital or visiting nurse who observed an entire breastfeeding.[7]

Hands-off Teaching

Many women do not appreciate having caregivers handle their breasts and babies. Weimers and colleagues explored the experience of Swedish mothers in receiving lactation assistance with their premature infants.[8] This research team was specifically interested in how women felt about the breastfeeding help they received, and they found that many women did not appreciate having their breasts touched by the helper. Several mothers reported feeling that their breasts were objectified by the helpers. The majority of mothers in that study found unexpected and unexplained hands-on assistance with breastfeeding to be unpleasant and unhelpful. This finding calls on lactation helpers to identify methods of helping mothers that do not include the helper handling the mother's breast and/or baby. The authors suggest a strategy of having the helper demonstrating positioning with a doll held in the helpers' arms.

Hoddinott and Pill also found that having breasts touched by professionals distressed some women in their sample.[9] This research team also identified a desire to have a professional talk them through good positioning or demonstrate it to them, rather than having the professional actually moving the breast or baby to achieve better latch.

Individualized Education

Women participating in Australian phenomenologic research stated that they did not want to receive standardized advice about feeding and problems. They felt that they had been helped when someone assessed their unique situation and gave individualized advice specific to their situation. In other words, women seek more of a coaching interaction than a standard educational exchange.[10]

A Woman-Centered Approach

Hoddinott and Pill found that mothers reported that care providers' words alone were insufficient.[11] They valued caregivers who spent time patiently watching them feed their baby. Women perceived that many caregivers valued continuation of breastfeeding above the contentedness and growth of their baby and were breastfeeding centered rather than woman centered.

Emotional and Concrete Support

Examining the experience of first-time mothers in Finland, Tarkka, Paunonen, and Laippala reported, "The greater the emotional and concrete support received by the mother from members of her support network, the better she coped with breastfeeding . . . Mothers who were upset while in the maternity ward coped less well with breastfeeding."[12]

Hong, Callister, and Schwartz explored the thoughts of first-time mothers, who valued most highly emotional and tangible support as well as good information. They identified unhelpful behaviors as hurried and/or inflexible care and failure to offer assistance with breastfeeding.[13]

■ The Needs of Adolescent Mothers

A qualitative study by Peterson, Sword, Charles, and DiCenso concerning the response of adolescent mothers to their postpartum care indicates that their satisfaction with care was strongly linked with the nurses' ability to place them at ease.[14] The authors write, "satisfactory experiences included nurses' sharing information about themselves, being calm, demonstrating confidence in mothers, speaking to adolescent and adult mothers in the same way, and anticipating unstated needs."[15]

Five common themes in the experience of adolescent mothers were identified by Dykes, Moran, Burt, and Edwards, including "feeling watched and judged, lacking confidence, tiredness, discomfort, and sharing accountability."[16] This research team went on to relate five support needs to the themes, "emotional support, esteem support, instrumental support, informational support, and network support."[17]

Self-esteem may be particularly at risk among adolescent mothers,[18] which indicates that care should be oriented to build the mother's sense of her ability to care for her little one.

■ Reaching out to the Mother

Unfortunately, women are often silent about their needs and expectations, particularly in interchanges with systems such as healthcare settings. Gill found that none of the mothers asked a nurse for help, even when experiencing difficulty.[19] If we are to discover the needs and wants of the breastfeeding women we serve, we must start by asking the true experts: the women themselves.

References

1. Raisler, J. (2000). Against the odds: Breastfeeding experiences of low income mothers. *Journal of Midwifery and Women's Health, 45*(3), 253–263.

2. Hoddinott, P., & Pill, R. (2000). A qualitative study of women's views about how health professionals communicate about infant feeding. *Health Expectations, 3*(4), 224.

3. Langer, A., Campero, L., Garcia, C., & Reynoso, S. (1998). Effects of psychosocial support during labour and childbirth on breastfeeding, medical interventions, and mothers' wellbeing in a Mexican public hospital: A randomised clinical trial. *British Journal of Obstetrics and Gynecology, 105*(10), 1056–1063.

4. Ekström, A., & Nissen, E. (2006). A mother's feelings for her infant are strengthened by excellent breastfeeding counseling and continuity of care. *Pediatrics, 118*(2), e309–e314.

5. Nelson, A. M. (2007). Maternal-newborn nurses' experiences of inconsistent professional breastfeeding support. *Journal of Advanced Nursing, 60*(1), 29–38.

6. Gill, S. L. (2001). The little things: Perceptions of breastfeeding support. *Journal of Obstetric, Gynecologic and Neonatal Nursing: JOGNN, 30*(4), 401–409.

7. Kuan, L. W., Britto, M., Decolongon, J., Schoettker, P. J., Atherton, H. D., & Kotagal, U. R. (1999). Health system factors contributing to breastfeeding success. *Pediatrics, 104*(3), e28.

8. Weimers, L., Svensson, K., Dumas, L., Navér, L., Wahlberg, V., et al. (2006). Hands-on approach during breastfeeding support in a neonatal intensive care unit: A qualitative study of Swedish mothers' experiences. *International Breastfeeding Journal, 26*(1), 20.

9. Hoddinott, P., & Pill, R. (2000). A qualitative study of women's views about how health professionals communicate about infant feeding. *Health Expectations, 3*(4), 224.

10. Hauck, Y., Langton, D., & Coyle, K. (2002). The path of determination: Exploring the lived experience of breastfeeding difficulties. *Breastfeeding Review, 10*(2), 5–12.

11. Hoddinott, P., & Pill, R. (2000). A qualitative study of women's views about how health professionals communicate about infant feeding. *Health Expectations, 3*(4), 224.

12. Tarkka, M. T., Paunonen, M., & Laippala, P. (1998). What contributes to breastfeeding success after childbirth in a maternity ward in Finland? *Birth, 25*(3), 175–181.

13. Hong, T. M., Callister, L. C., & Schwartz, R. (2003). First time mothers' views of breastfeeding support from nurses. *MCN: The American Journal of Maternal Child Nursing, 28*(1), 10–5.

14. Peterson, W. E., Sword, W., Charles, C., & DiCenso, A. (2007). Adolescents' perceptions of inpatient postpartum nursing care. *Qualitative Health Research, 17*(2), 201–212.

15. Peterson, W. E., Sword, W., Charles, C., & DiCenso, A. (2007). Adolescents' perceptions of inpatient postpartum nursing care. *Qualitative Health Research, 17*(2), 201.

16. Dykes, F., Moran, V. H., Burt, S., & Edwards, J. (2003). Adolescent mothers and breastfeeding: Experiences and support needs—an exploratory study. *Journal of Human Lactation, 19*(4), 391–401.

17. Dykes, F., Moran, V. H., Burt, S., & Edwards, J. (2003). Adolescent mothers and breastfeeding: Experiences and support needs—an exploratory study. *Journal of Human Lactation, 19*(4), 391.

18. McVeigh, C., & Smith, M. (2000). A comparison of adult and teenage mothers' self-esteem and satisfaction with social support. *Midwifery, 16*(4), 269–276.

19. Gill, S. L. (2001). The little things: Perceptions of breastfeeding support. *Journal of Obstetric, Gynecologic and Neonatal Nursing: JOGNN, 30*(4), 401–409.

CHAPTER

13

Improving Maternity Care for Breastfeeding Through Practice Change

For many years practitioners and researchers focused their energy on trying to understand the women who choose breastfeeding and have breastfeeding experiences they would describe as optimal. What are their ages compared to women who don't breastfeed? Are they better educated? Do they have more financial or social resources? Do they have other demographic indicators in common? Eventually the understanding emerged that it wasn't so much the type of woman that determined optimal breastfeeding outcomes, it was the prenatal, maternity care and community policies and practices she encountered. The good news is that although we can't make a mother more affluent or older or better educated, we can change our policies and practices.

■ Practice Change is the Key to Improving Outcomes

Several research studies have shown that implementation of the practices described in the *Ten Steps to Successful Breastfeeding*, which form the core of the WHO/UNICEF Baby-Friendly Hospital Initiative (BFHI), improve breastfeeding outcomes. The most compelling is probably the Promotion of Breastfeeding Intervention Trial (PROBIT). Kramer and others[1] conducted this cluster-randomized trial in the Republic of Belarus in order to determine how health provider and healthcare system practices could change breastfeeding duration and exclusivity and health outcomes among children in the first year. PROBIT was a large study (17,046 mother/infant pairs) of full-term singleton infants weighing at least 2500 g and their healthy mothers who intended to breastfeed. Almost 97% of the participants were followed for the entire year of the study.

Sixteen sites were randomized to receive the experimental intervention modeled on the *Ten Steps to Successful Breastfeeding*. These sites experienced new breastfeeding policies, training, and support to change practices in support of breastfeeding. The fifteen control sites were randomized to continue their usual infant feeding practices and policies.

The outcomes of the PROBIT trial showed that all of the measurements of breastfeeding duration at 12 months (intervention group 19.7%; control group 11.4%) and exclusive breastfeeding at 3 months (intervention group 43.3%; control group 6.4%) and at 6 months (intervention group 7.9%; control group 0.6%) were significantly higher at the intervention sites compared to the control sites. In addition, there was a significant reduction in the risk of 1 or more gastro-intestinal tract infections (9.1% in the intervention group; 13.2% in the control group) and of atopic eczema (intervention group, 3.3%; control group, 6.3%), but no significant reduction in respiratory tract infection (intervention group, 39.2%; control group, 39.4%).

In a study of the effects of early contact, suckling, and rooming-in on infant abandonment, Lvoff, Lvoff, and Klaus found that implementation of the Baby-Friendly Hospital Initiative almost halved the rate of abandonment. The mean *decreased* from 50.3 +/- 5.8 per 10,000 births in the first 6 years to 27.8 +/- 8.7 per 10,000 births in the next 6 years. A similar hospital had a 32% *increase* over the same time period.[2]

DiGirolamo, Grummer-Strawn, and Fein[3] examined a U.S. nationwide sample of more than 1000 women who intended to breastfeed for at least 2 months. The research measured the exposure of the mothers to practices not in keeping with the *Ten Steps to Successful Breastfeeding*, such as pacifier use, supplementation, not rooming-in, scheduled feedings, and getting off to a late start at breastfeeding. They found that although pacifier use was the most prevalent practice (more than 68% of the mothers had been given pacifiers for their babies while in the hospital), supplementation had the most negative effect on breastfeeding outcomes, with getting off to a late start as the other negative effect. When the researchers examined the effect of the combination of helpful practices, they found that the more helpful practices that the mother experienced, the more likely she was to have made it to her goal of breastfeeding for at least 2 months (please see Figure 13-1).

What's the conclusion? Practice change is the key to changing breastfeeding and child health outcomes. Please see Box 13-1.

■ Quality Improvement— A Proven Strategy for Practice Change

The use of quality improvement (QI) and quality improvement tools has been widely shown to be effective in changing the practices that improve patient outcomes and optimize healthcare delivery. As a result, QI has been well accepted in the healthcare setting and considered key to delivering optimal patient care. Maternity care practices and policies related to breastfeeding are ideally suited to quality focused strategies; quality tools are ideal for examining practices and monitoring breastfeeding policies and protocols that support, protect, and promote breastfeeding.

Targets for breastfeeding have been set nationally and they can form the beginning goals for maternity care settings and their communities. Then, work should be focused in order to improve the rates of breastfeeding initiation, exclusivity, and duration on the institution and community level. If fewer women leave the hospital breastfeeding than intended to on admission, this information can also be used as the beginning of the quality project. A bonus is that accrediting agencies support the use of QI tools to examine and change patient care practices.

■ Quality Improvement Didn't Begin in Healthcare Settings

During the 1980s, the Deming management method[4] evolved into quality improvement programs for industry and took on many

> **Box 13-1**
>
> Practice change is the key to changing breastfeeding and child health outcomes.

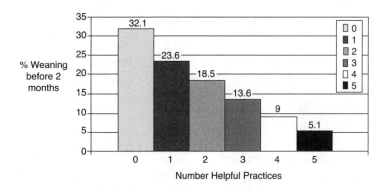

Figure 13-1 The effect of increased helpful breastfeeding practices on weaning before two months. *Source*: Adapted from DiGirolamo, et al.

names and variations: continuous quality management (CQM), total quality improvement (TQI), and others. Success in industry and other customer service sectors came first, then hospitals began engaging in the quality improvement process. They found that patient satisfaction increased as quality improvement increased. Hospitals found that it was possible to engineer dramatic improvements in quality of care through systematic intervention.[5]

■ With QI, Data Is the Driver

A fundamental difference between QI and other change models is the belief that *data* drives improvement. Without measurement, strategies become activity driven rather than results driven.[6] Meaningful, ongoing data provides the hard evidence that is needed to make unbiased change. In a QI environment, individual units or cross-disciplinary teams of hospital staff members and community representatives are able to identify problems and use QI tools and practices to improve the delivery of care as related to breastfeeding and other health behaviors.

Because the underpinning of QI is total dedication to the customer, the first question the breastfeeding QI team must ask itself is, "Who is our customer?" As Widström and Righard have so dramatically demonstrated in video, the baby is the customer.[7,8] Widström succinctly summarized the construct: "breastfeeding is the baby's choice." Babies want to be near their mother, be warm, hear their mothers' heartbeat, and nurse after they are born, but hospital practices may interfere with the process. The principles of QI dictate that "all activities of all functions are designed and carried out so that all

requirements of all the ultimate customers are met and expectations exceeded."[9] This point of view, applied to the baby who ardently desires to be breastfed, dictates that staff practices and the organization of care are designed to strive toward the ultimate outcome of an effectively nursing baby.[10]

When selecting projects to address in quality improvement studies, the QI team should choose those projects that have the following:

- a high impact on quality and cost
- practice patterns that can be changed
- measurable outcomes

A basic component of QI is the use of various tools to do the following:

- examine and point to the root causes of problems
- state these problems clearly and diagrammatically
- develop and implement strategies to decrease and, ultimately, eliminate the problem

This paradigm expects excellence. It is not acceptable that *some* babies are discharged having latched on and are nursing well. Excuses are not accepted. Blame is not levied. Data is collected and improvements are tried. Outcomes are evaluated, barriers and solutions are identified, and the practice is improved again.

■ Start by Making a Process Map

We find it helpful to begin a quality improvement journey by developing a *process map or process audit*—a visual representation of the steps or activities that are performed. Process mapping allows everyone involved to do the following:

- visualize what is going on
- assess the current situation
- examine the external environment (those things that seem uncontrollable such as which services are reimbursable or rates of reimbursement)
- examine the internal environment (those things that are under their direct control)

- chart what they want for their future environment
- develop a performance improvement plan that will improve the quality of the services they offer to breastfeeding women

In a process audit, the QI team is mapping the path (the process) of a selected item or person. In Figure 13-2, this will be the mother and also the baby. It could alternately

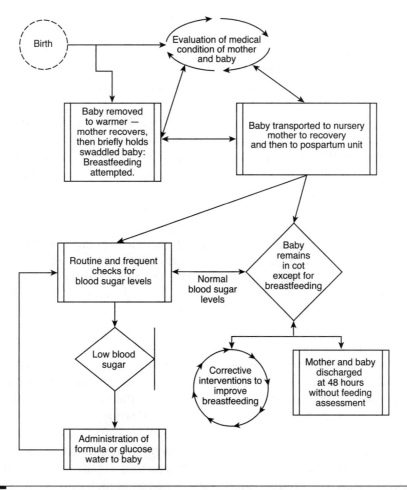

Figure 13-2 Example of Process Audit which Optimally Supports the Ten Steps to Successful Breastfeeding.
Source: © Healthy Children Project. Used with Permission.

be a client, a nurse, a physician, midwife, or other healthcare provider. Then, the team overlays the mother and baby's process in a visual way so that the team can see and understand the process. They would do this with a number of mother/baby pairs to capture individual variations, but are warned not to get too caught up in detail.

Figure 13-2 is a map of an audit that was done in a hospital with poor breastfeeding outcomes. In this hospital, 62% of breastfed babies were supplemented (with formula or glucose water) without medical cause, and about half (51%) of the mothers had stopped breastfeeding by 2 months. For 1 week during the process audit, all mothers and babies were followed, and the map was drawn to reflect the path of most of the mothers and babies in the audit.

The audit map starts at the birth because mothers who give birth in this hospital rarely attended childbirth or breastfeeding classes, although they may have come during pregnancy for a hospital tour or orientation. Some mothers had attended a prenatal breastfeeding session at a nutrition support program, but it was not associated with the hospital and did not cover labor, birth, or the hospital stay in regard to breastfeeding.

Babies, once born, are weighed, wiped off, and examined away from the mother in a warmer. The mother is evaluated separately. Once the staff completes the assessment, procedures, and paperwork, the baby is wrapped and offered to the mother to hold. She is asked if she wants to try breastfeeding. But the baby breastfeeds best after a period of continuous skin-to-skin with the mother, and when wrapped is not ready to breastfeed. Staff then remove the baby to the nursery and

the mother is transported to a postpartum room. More breastfeeding attempts follow, but the baby spends the time in between attempts in the cot either in the mother's room or in the nursery. Glucose checks indicate that about 20% of breastfed babies in this hospital are thought to have low blood sugar levels and are given glucose water or formula as a result. The other 42% of breastfed babies who are given formula are considered too sleepy to breastfeed, won't latch on, or cry at the breast, or their mothers are too tired to breastfeed them.

The nurse responsible for discharge teaching reviews the mother's and baby's charts prior to discharge and tries to teach the mother how to overcome her breastfeeding difficulties. She encourages the mother to get breastfeeding help in the community after going home.

The process map shown in Figure 13-3 reflects an audit of a hospital that was implementing a fairly effective strategy in support of breastfeeding.

Notice that this hospital reached into the prenatal community with breastfeeding education. It did this by partnering with the obstetricians and midwives whose clients would give birth in the hospital. The hospital breastfeeding committee developed a checklist of discussion topics to be covered with each mother during the prenatal visits. They also conducted on-site in-service meetings for the office staff so that they would be oriented to the new hospital breastfeeding policies and be prepared to teach and respond to mothers' questions.

During labor, mothers are encouraged to move around and walk, eat lightly, and have the companion or companions of their

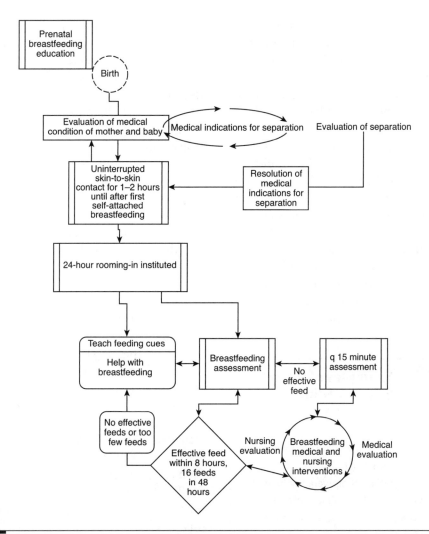

Figure 13-3 Example of an Ineffective Process for Supporting Breastfeeding in a Sample Hospital.
Source: © Healthy Children Project. Used with Permission.

choice with them at all times. After the birth, the baby is dried off and placed skin to skin on the mother's chest where it remains, uninterrupted (except if a medical problem is discovered), until the first breastfeeding has been finished. For mothers who have given birth via a cesarean section, the baby is placed

skin to skin with the mother as soon as she is able to respond, which, since general anesthesia is rarely used, she is ordinarily able to do as soon as she would be for a vaginal birth. The baby and mother are evaluated while in skin-to-skin contact, and the baby is footprinted, banded, and given vitamin K and eye care as well. If there are medical indications for separation of mother and baby, skin-to-skin contact is initiated as soon as they are reunited.

Twenty-four-hour rooming-in is the norm for all mothers in this facility, and it is initiated after the first breastfeed. Mothers are taught about feeding cues, encouraged to feed on cue, and that the baby should end the feeding. All of the staff on the postpartum unit have been trained to assess breastfeedings, and each mother/baby dyad is assessed at least once every 8 hours. Whenever a feeding is deemed ineffective, the baby is observed for feeding cues, and the next feeding is observed with coaching of corrective interventions by the staff. The staff has the expectation that there will be at least 16 effective feedings in

the first 48 hours. Most mothers have 20 or more feedings prior to discharge. In this hospital, there is an integration of medical and nursing evaluations with the breastfeeding assessments.

A Pareto analysis is the process of ranking QI opportunities in order to determine which projects should be pursued first. Pareto offers a way to separate all of the possible issues into manageable QI projects. Potential indicators are listed in Box 13-2. The indicators are written to capture the percentage of mothers and babies who are *not* receiving optimal practices that promote and support breastfeeding. Other helpful QI tools include fishbone or Ishikawa diagrams and C charts.

By using QI tools and strategies, the QI team can ascertain what information they have that defines the problem and what information they have that differentiates the problem from what ought to be happening, and they can think about what the situation would look like without a problem.

Through performance analysis, the QI team can answer the questions, "Why aren't we delivering excellent practice?" and "What's getting in the way of excellent practice?" Then they can ask, "What does the literature say about barriers to success for this problem?"

| **Box 13-2** | **Examples of Hospital Breastfeeding Indicators** |

What percentage of babies were not held skin to skin for at least the first hour?

What percentage of mothers were not helped with breastfeeding in the first hour?

What percentage of babies were not exclusively breastfed at discharge?

What percentage of babies were not nursing well at 8 hours?

What percentage of babies are not rooming in 24 hours a day?

What percentage of mothers do not go to childbirth or breastfeeding classes?

What percentage of mothers do not utilize community mother-to-mother support?

■ In Our Experience . . .

We have spent many years working with staff determined to change hospital practices to be more supportive of breastfeeding. In our experience, some strategies seem to be more effective than others, so we'd like discuss them and make some recommendations.

- Get an interdisciplinary committee together and fill out the Baby-Friendly self-appraisal tool. Download the tool from babyfriendlyusa.org. The tool serves as a great discussion outline. Don't expect to get through the whole tool in one session with a group, even though you could read it through and fill it out in less than an hour.

- Circulate a newsletter (online is fine) that informs everyone about the committee's work. One hospital started with a committee of only four faithful attendees, but it sent its newsletter out to everyone who routinely cared for mothers or babies. Over the time span of a few years, attendance grew to 40 and the hospital had to change to a larger meeting room. Another facility focused its newsletter on one practice change a month, such as skin-to-skin contact, rooming-in, and so on.

- Use the hospital email to increase interest in your projects. One hospital did this with a quiz question posted each day.

- Discover what other projects your hospital has committed to or is currently working on. How are these projects being managed? What is the impetus behind the commitment? How is your project similar to these? By pointing out similarities, you may more effectively engage administration.

- Start by making the rule that evidence will be used to determine practice, and decide on the hierarchy of evidence that will be adhered to by the committee. Hospitals that use evidence to make decisions and could be characterized as learning organizations are more likely to use evidence to make decisions about breastfeeding support practices rather than be content with the way they have always done it.

- Value effective teamwork. We have noted that breastfeeding divas are singularly ineffective in moving forward change. Instead, interdisciplinary committees led by credible champions are successful.

- Tackle the easiest steps first. We know it seems counterintuitive since some steps may look like they will take a long time and you might think you should tackle them first, but remember, nothing feeds success like success.

- Consider creating posters on the unit to track progress visually.

- Celebrate all the time! Have a party for every mark of progress.

- Engage the quality department to participate in measuring performance.

- Engage the medical librarian to provide the compelling research studies that are needed to make evidence-based practice change.

- Assure support from the highest levels of leadership. In some cases this has been a member of the board of directors, the president of the hospital corporation, or the director of marketing.

- Break projects into their smallest components and be willing to make incremental changes. Baby steps add up!

- Don't discount impatience as a positive feature of your work! Being happy with the way you have always done it is the alternative, and that gets you nowhere!

- If your committee isn't working well as a team, consider bringing in a facilitator. We have found that committees are most successful if the breastfeeding expert does *not* take a position of leadership. This is the role of the champion, but if that doesn't work, a facilitator is better than having the breastfeeding expert take the leadership role. This technique allows the breastfeeding expert the latitude to speak up rather than conducting the meetings.

- At an early meeting, make decisions about the following questions:
  - What are our goals?
  - How will data be collected?
  - What changes within the organization will need to be made?
  - How will we be able to measure change?
  - How will the data be collected?
  - What hierarchy of evidence will be used?

- Steer away from blaming and finger pointing. It's easy to think that the problem is the mothers, the night shift, the doctors, management, or anyone but us! When fingers are pointed, change doesn't happen.

We have seen hospitals become so facile in making changes around breastfeeding practices that the members of the breastfeeding committee went on to become the change agents for other practices not related to breastfeeding.

We wish you a smooth path in your work to improve health outcomes for mothers and babies through practice change.

References

1. Kramer, M. S., Chalmers, B., Hodnett, E. D., Sevkovskaya, Z., Dzikovich, I., Shapiro, S., et al., for the PROBIT Study Group (Promotion of Breastfeeding Intervention Trial). (2001, January 24–31). Promotion of Breastfeeding Intervention Trial (PROBIT): A randomized trial in the Republic of Belarus. *Journal of the American Medical Association, 285*(4), 413–420.
2. Lvoff, N. M., Lvoff, V., & Klaus, N. H. (2000). Effect of the baby-friendly initiative on infant abandonment in a Russian hospital. *Archives of Pediatric and Adolescent Medicine, 154,* 474–477.
3. DiGirolamo, A. M., Grummer-Strawn, L. M., & Fein, S. (2001). Maternity care practices: Implications for breastfeeding. *Birth, 28*(2), 94–100.
4. Walton, M. (1991). *The Deming Management Method.* New York: Putnam.
5. Lebov, W. & Scott, G. (1992). *Service Quality Improvement: The Customer Satisfaction Strategy for Health Care.* Chicago: American Hospital Publishing, p. 9.
6. Schaffer, R. H. & Thomas, H. A. (1992). Successful change programs begin with results. *Harvard Business Review, 70,* 80.
7. Widström, A. M. (2007). *Breastfeeding is Baby's Choice* [DVD]. Available from www.health education.cc.
8. Righard, L. (1992). *Delivery Self Attachment* [DVD]. Sunland, CA: Geddes Productions.
9. Ciampa, D. (1991). *Total Quality: A User's Guide for Implementation.* Reading, MA: Addison-Wesley, p. 6.
10. Cadwell, K. (1997). Using the quality improvement process to affect breastfeeding protocols in United States Hospitals. *Journal of Human Lactation, 13,* 5.

Index

Note: *f* = figure; *t* = table

A

AAP. *See* American Academy of Pediatrics
Abandonment, of infant, 150
Abandonment of breastfeeding
    due to unresolved problems, 62, 120
    late breastfeeding initiative and, 136
    pacifier use and, 111
    risk factors for, 60, 62
Academy of Breastfeeding Medicine (ABM)
    peripartum breastfeeding management, 53, 54, 55
    supplemental feeding protocol, 113
    teaching and postpartum assessment content, 64
ACOG (American College of Obstetricians and
    Gynecologists), 53–55
Adolescent mothers, needs of, 147
Advice for mother
    consistent, 64
    inconsistent, 65
Agency for Healthcare Research and Quality (AHRQ), 20
American Academy of Pediatrics (AAP)
    evaluation of breastfeeding, 62
    feeding adequacy assessment, 121
    pacifier use, SIDS risk and, 112
    peripartum breastfeeding policy, 53, 54, 55

American College of Obstetricians and Gynecologists
    (ACOG), 53–55
Assessment
    barriers to, 65–68
    of feeding adequacy, 121
    of hospital feedings, 60
    Mother-Baby, 66, 67
    need for, 58
    tools for, 65–67
At-breast feeders, 109
At-breast supplementers, 113
Attachment behavior, immediate skin-to-skin contact and,
    52–53
Attitude change, from staff training, 28, 31
Audit process
    for breastfeeding committee, 103
    for breastfeeding on demand, 101
    for maternal-baby separation, 86
    for rooming-in, 88–89
Australian posture, 60
Authorities, belief in without evidence, 13

B

Babe cafés, 120
Babies Were Born to Be Breastfed campaign, 38
Baby-Friendly Hospital Initiative (BFHI), 129–138